D1249793

ALSO BY MICHELLE HARRISON

A Woman in Residence

Self-Help for Premenstrual Syndrome

New and Revised

Michelle Harrison, M.D.

Self-Help for Premenstrual Syndrome

New and Revised

Random House New York

Copyright © 1982 by Michelle Harrison

All rights reserved under International and Pan-American Copyright Conventions.
Published in the United States by Random House, Inc., New York, and
simultaneously in Canada by Random House of Canada Limited, Toronto.
This edition was originally published by Matrix Press in 1982.

Library of Congress Cataloging in Publication Data

Harrison, Michelle.
Self-help for premenstrual syndrome.

1. Premenstrual syndrome. 2. Self-care, Health.
I. Title. II. Title: Self-help for pre-menstrual syndrome.
RG165.H37   1985   618.1'72   84-23723
ISBN 0-394-73502-1

Manufactured in the United States of America

24689753

FIRST EDITION

To Heather, Abigail, and Cecilia

Acknowledgments

―――――――――――※―――――――――――

Books are eventually born, after lengthy and at times troublesome gestations, involving many people's thoughts and hands. Such has been the history of this book, now more fully developed and expanded from its first emergence in December 1982.

The following people have shared in its creation.

Bobbi Ausubel, Tom Brennen, Claire Boskin, Kathy Burke, Gray Cahill, Patti Cannon, Virginia Cassara, Mary Catherine, Savitri Clarke, Judy Coons, Marian Copeland, Belita Cowan, Katherina Dalton, Jody Dupuis, Lee Erhartic, Vicki Gabriner, Eva Graf, Andrea Halliday, Jean Hamilton, Beth Horning, Ruth Hubbard, Mary Kate Jordan, Linda Kennedy, Gail Koplow, Lindsay Leckie, Molly Lovelock, Mary Lowry, Barbara Macdonald, Charlotte Mayerson, Susanne Morgan, Ann Murphy, Ronald Norris, Judy Norsigian, Monica Raymond, Wendy Sanford, Prilly Sanville, Ellie Siegel, Sybil Shainwald, Marjorie Snyder, Jerry Whiting and Laura Zimmerman.

A special thanks to Patricia Carrington, who provided clarity and reassurance at the end.

And to Shirley Yetz, who warmly provided secretarial help and enthusiastic care of the baby.

And to my parents, Emily and David Alman, and my sister, Jenny Michaels, who continue to support my marching to a slightly different drummer.

Contents

PART I: What Is PMS?

CHAPTER	1	Introduction	*3*
CHAPTER	2	The PMS Dilemma	*6*
CHAPTER	3	The Many Symptoms of PMS	*10*
CHAPTER	4	Causes of PMS	*25*
CHAPTER	5	Premenstrual Magnification (PMM)	*30*
CHAPTER	6	Diagnosis	*33*

PART II: Treatment of PMS

CHAPTER	7	Treatment of PMS	*75*
CHAPTER	8	Diet and PMS	*78*
CHAPTER	9	Exercise	*88*
CHAPTER	10	Stress and PMS	*94*
CHAPTER	11	Vitamins, Minerals, and Oil of Evening Primrose	*103*
CHAPTER	12	Progesterone	*107*
CHAPTER	13	Antiprostaglandins, Antidepressants and Diuretics	*116*
CHAPTER	14	Acupuncture and Other Alternative Therapies	*120*
CHAPTER	15	Psychotherapy	*124*
CHAPTER	16	Support Groups	*126*

PART III: Broader Aspects of PMS

CHAPTER 17   Sexuality and PMS *133*
CHAPTER 18   The Family and PMS *139*
CHAPTER 19   Creativity and PMS *148*
CHAPTER 20   Social and Political Implications *150*
CHAPTER 21   Getting Help for PMS *155*

           Selected Bibliography *161*
           Cookbooks *165*
           Resources for Books and Tapes *167*
           Food Sources *169*
           PMS Resources *171*
           Blank Charts *173*

PART I

❖

What Is PMS?

CHAPTER 1

Introduction

HOW DO I KNOW THAT PMS EXISTS?
Medically it is a striking phenomenon. In my medical practice, at lectures and through the mail, thousands of women have told me such things as: "I'm not me that time of the month"; "My body swells up and I look like I'm pregnant. My rings and shoes get tight"; "When I'm premenstrual the least little thing makes me cry"; "I just want to be alone and hide until I get my period"; "I can't go back to school because when I'm premenstrual I can't focus on the page"; "Getting my period is a bother, but being premenstrual is a nightmare."

As a child I remember women sitting around a neighbor's kitchen table talking about irritability at that time of month, eating ice cream and potato chips at that time of the month, and dealing with husbands and children at that time of month. They weren't talking about menstruation, for that had other words like "having my friend" or "getting" it, said with a raising of one or both eyebrows that let everyone know what was meant.

It is clear that PMS exists because among the thousands of women I have listened to I have *never* had one say that each month, *after* her period, she loses self-esteem or fights with her husband or wants to kill herself. I've never heard a woman say that she wanted to feel *postmenstrually* as well as she does each month premenstrually. I've never heard a woman say, "You know, I get irritated easily, but premenstrually nothing could bother me." Whatever this phenomenon is, it appears to occur only premenstrually. Yes, women have difficulties other times of the month, but for those whose problems occur in relation to their menstrual cycles, they are always reported as occurring premenstrually.

I'm struck by the diversity of the women I see: women in positions of power, who hold responsible jobs, but for whom PMS is a private agony; women living in poverty with three children still in diapers who premenstrually struggle against their bodies and their living conditions to maintain a sense order and hope.

In 1982 I wrote of my feelings about PMS:

> *How do I feel about PMS? I am conflicted. The feminist in me wishes that our biology were irrelevant. The doctor in me sees the need for recognizing and treating premenstrual symptoms. The woman in me recognizes the power of the biological forces within me, and wishes I lived in a society in which my menstrual cycle were seen as an asset, not a liability. The writer in me keeps hoping that if I can get it all down on paper, it will be easier to understand, and in any case, I will not be alone in my dilemma or my conflict.*

Today I remain conflicted, but I see the problem in a slightly different way. When I see the dramatic effect of dietary change on many, many women's PMS, then I think to myself: Something terrible is happening to women in our society. I wonder if we are somehow being destroyed by what we routinely eat and how we live. And when I look at women struggling with their PMS through life-style changes or medications, I ask why this is happening.

Is it possible that there are lessons for women *and* men in PMS? Is the greater sensitivity experienced by women premenstrually something we all, as a society, need to learn about? Without wanting to glorify or romanticize their pain, I wonder what growth will come to women as they confront PMS. What would the world be like if men sometimes seemed to cry without reason? What would we then believe about vulnerability or sensitivity?

Are there lessons regarding responsibility, anger, or violence, to be learned from PMS, lessons applicable to both men and to women? I wonder how we will look at PMS in twenty years? What will we have learned, and most importantly, how will we be dealing responsibly and compassionately with that knowledge?

Our strength as women must lie in our honesty and in our commitment to help each other, to concentrate on the ways we are more like each other than different. To these ends, we must continue to explore the cyclic nature of our lives, recognizing both its strengths and vulnerabilities, while remembering that our expressions and aspirations are still limited by a society in which we have not yet achieved equality.

This book examines the physical and emotional symptoms of PMS, their origins, and ways to deal with them. To present this information, I have drawn on my work as a physician who specializes in PMS, on the research that is available, and on traditional as well as nontraditional treatments that I have found to be effective.

Much work remains to be done on PMS. Women and their healers must try to share what they know. I hope this book will have a place in that process.

CHAPTER 2

The PMS Dilemma

"YOU KNOW YOU'LL FEEL BETTER when your period starts." Hours later, Alex's words still reverberated in Sally's head, making clear thought or action impossible. Behind the closed door of her office, she sat at her desk, twisting paper clips and crumpling tiny pieces of tissue paper.

In the minutes before leaving home that morning, Sally had said she was ending her marriage. She felt that she was at the end of caring, the end of giving, and had screamed at Alex that it was all over, that she wanted him to leave, that she couldn't stand living with him anymore. With a sinking feeling she realized that Amanda, their three-year-old, had heard the entire battle. She clutched the child and quickly left the house with her. Stopping briefly at the day-care center, she told the teachers that Amanda might be upset and then guiltily went on to work.

Driving along the river, gliding in and out of slow and faster lanes, she experienced confusion, despair, and anger. She wasn't sure of who she was, what she was feeling, or why. The driving helped her, creating the distance she needed now in her struggle for inner clarity.

Mornings were always the worst, when she woke to find herself between the fading darkness and dreams. Sally needed to be alone when she awakened, to gather slowly the strength for the demands which seemed to drain her. That need seemed especially strong this morning. She had awakened feeling bloated, wanting to hold on to the darkness that hid the distortions of her body, kept her from the mirror and skirt snaps that were the enemies of her self-esteem. Her skin had crawled, and she had thought that if only the world would leave her alone, she might just make it through.

Work was a different world. Here, where she managed the production department of a major trade publication, she competently made decisions, negotiated, managed people and policies. Here her life with Alex seemed unreal. Shuffling papers, trying to overcome her despair, she fought the intruding thought: was her marriage over?

Had Alex been right? That question, one she sometimes asked herself and sometimes fled, now left her feeling sick, vulnerable, naked. *If this were a week from now, would she feel better?* After her period arrived, would she simply smile and say she must have been tired? Would the rage, confusion, desperate need to be alone have vanished?

Does Sally have *premenstrual syndrome?* Will she be all right when her period starts? Which is the real Sally? Is she out of control premenstrually, or is she simply suppressing her real feelings the rest of the month? Does Sally have an illness, as is implied by the word "syndrome," or is she experiencing the mood shifts that are a normal part of everyone's life?

What about other women? What about women who have a day of blues premenstrually? What about women who are premenstrually suicidal or unable to function? Are those states all separate conditions or points on a continuum, and at what point is it "illness"?

In the past fifty years we have seen the increasing medicalization of women's normal functions. Childbirth has become a technological event, often a surgical procedure. Menopause is often seen as a disease to be treated, frequently in the face of the woman's protest that she feels fine and doesn't want medication.

Women's expressions of strong emotions have historically been labeled as medical disease. Women who have been emotional or angry have been treated with hysterectomies, lobotomies, shock therapy, and tranquilizers.

And what about women who lead lives of constant stress, centered on poverty and on trying to feed children? If those women feel out of control or despairing one week of the month, do we call that illness? How much stress should someone be able to bear?

In looking at illness, Western culture traditionally tends to split the body from the mind, to see the two as distinct entities, often unrelated to each other. If we define a disease as physical, then we are not "responsible" for it. If it is emotional, then we not only assign blame for its development (parents have done it to us, etc.) but are also held responsible for overcoming it. We tend to believe that physical disease happens to us and that mental disease we bring on ourselves.

In recent years medicine has given more attention to the intricate interplay between body and mind. Heart disease and cancer are physical diseases that have been shown to be strongly influenced, if not caused, by environment, diet, stress, and personality dynamics. Depression, an emotional disorder, also has physical manifestations, including at times biochemical changes now measurable with laboratory testing. Whether the biochemical change is a cause or a result of the depression remains unanswered. Women living in dormitories unknowingly begin to synchronize their menstrual cycles. Testosterone levels in males are altered by their positions of dominance. Hormones can produce emotional changes and social interactions can elicit hormonal changes.

Premenstrual syndrome is usually described as a disorder either of body (advocates of that theory believe there is a basic biological flaw in a large percentage of women of reproductive age) or of mind (a woman with PMS has not "accepted her role as a woman"). The issue of whether PMS is physical or mental becomes further polarized because of the significance we place on whether we can define an illness as physical or emotional. But in fact all diseases raise this issue. PMS is just one more example.

Physicians said for years that dysmenorrhea, severe menstrual cramps, were due to a woman's ambivalence about womanhood. When prostaglandins were discovered to be related to the cramping, this theory lost favor, but in the meantime generations of women were treated as though this belief were fact. Women were told they had cramps because they didn't like being women, that they were "rejecting the feminine role."

Our culture has a negative attitude toward menstruation. That there are women who report increased efficiency, creativity, and sensitivity during their premenstrual times, sometimes even in the presence of uncomfortable physical or emotional states, has received little if any attention in the medical literature. It is often difficult for professionals to hear what women are really saying, and thus even the research can be tainted by personal biases. For example, attempts are currently being made to separate what women "really" feel from what they "think" they feel, a distinction that implies a certain deafness to what is being said and an assumption that there is a difference between the two.

It is imperative that as we look at PMS, we allow for open questioning, that we examine our own biases, the difference between what we want PMS to be and what women who suffer with it tell us it *is*. At the same time we must also remain sensitive and responsive to how this knowledge will be heard and used by a society that is often biased against women's interpretations of truth.

CHAPTER 3

⊠

The Many Symptoms
of PMS

ALL THE SYMPTOMS OF PMS can occur as part of other illnesses or other life experiences. What characterizes them as PMS is their **cyclicity,** their persistent, repetitive occurrence on a monthly basis prior to menstruation. Having one or even a few of these symptoms does not necessarily mean that you are ill, but being *incapacitated* by them does.

> *Approximately fifteen days after the start of my monthly period I find myself with complete lack of interest in life in general. I have problems with vision, and craving for food. I become anxious, lose interest in sex. This started three years ago and became gradually worse with time. After fourteen days I am back to normal. My doctor calls it nerves, but when I ask him why it lasts fourteen days and hits me the same time every month, he shakes his head and leaves the room. One of his thoughts is that most women need more sex.*
>
> *My husband is so sensitive to my feelings he will say to me, "It started again. I can tell by the expression on your face. You don't have to hide it. I only wish I could help."*

Any of the following symptoms may occur premenstrually as part of PMS:

Abdominal bloating
Abdominal cramping
Absentmindedness
Accident-proneness
Acne
Alcohol intolerance
Anger
Anxiety
Asthma
Back pain
Breast swelling and pain
Cardiac arrhythmias (irregular heartbeats)
Confusion
Crying
Depression
Dizziness
Eating disorders
Edema
Eye difficulties
Fainting
Fatigue
Food binges
Hand tingling and numbness
Headaches
Hemorrhoids (flare-ups)
Herpes (oral, skin, genital)
Hives
Indecisiveness
Infections
Insomnia

Irritability
Joint swelling and pain
Lack of coordination
Lactation difficulties
Lethargy
Muscle aches
Nausea
Noise sensitivity
Palpitations (heart pounding)
Panic states
Paranoia
Pimple eruptions
Rashes
Salt cravings
Seizures
Self-esteem (lack thereof)
Sex-drive changes
Slurred speech
Smell sensitivity
Spaciness
Stiff neck
Styes
Suicidal thoughts
Sweet cravings
Tension
Tiredness
Touch sensitivity
Urinary difficulties
Violence
Weight gain
Withdrawal

The Cycle Is the Link

The actual symptoms of PMS in this list are generally considered non-specific—that is, they are not indicative of any one cause, but may result from many different disorders. For instance, headache may be caused by allergy, hypoglycemia (low blood sugar), chemical toxins, tension, brain tumors, stress, nutritional disorders, etc. Fatigue may be caused by anemia, stress, vitamin deficiency, etc. The *timing* of the symptoms determines whether a woman has PMS. For example, the fatigue of PMS occurs *only* premenstrually. If it is caused by anemia, a woman will feel fatigued all month. Generally, premenstrual symptoms begin some time after ovulation and end with menstruation.

Characteristics of PMS Symptoms

- They may be mild and hardly noticeable to severe and incapacitating.
- They begin at some time between ovulation and menstruation.
- They may last one or two days to two weeks. In some cases, over time, they spread into the postmenstrual days so that there may be only one week or so left in which there are no symptoms.
- They may occur at any time in a woman's life, from menarche (the time of the first menstrual period) to past menopause.
- They tend to increase in severity with age.
- They may occur after a hysterectomy, with or without removal of ovaries.
- They may occur after tubal ligation or even after tubal or ovarian surgery.
- They may occur after severe illnesses or major physical, emotional, or sexual traumas.
- They may occur some months and not others.
- They may be more severe some months than others.
- There is usually some consistency to the symptoms but at times the specific symptoms may vary from month to month.
- Each month with the onset of menses or shortly thereafter symptoms leave, often abruptly.

How the Physical Symptoms Are Experienced

ABDOMINAL BLOATING, JOINT SWELLING, EDEMA (GENERALIZED WATER RETENTION):

> *I feel as if I have gained a hundred pounds and I can barely tolerate my children. I feel as if I am going to jump out of my skin.*

> *Nothing fits, and I sometimes think that if I stuck a*
> *pin in my body all this water would pour out.*

Premenstrually water may collect in the tissues of the abdomen as well as in the ankles, other joints, and in the face. Although some women do gain weight during this time (as much as ten to twelve pounds each month), what is actually happening is that body fluids are being redistributed. Some women experience an increase in thirst. Others have a characteristic puffiness around their eyes. There are models and actresses who try to avoid having photographs taken at that time because of the change in their appearance. You may need to wear larger clothes premenstrually because of abdominal bloating. Many women complain that they have to keep two sizes of clothing to wear at different times in their cycles. Your shoes may feel tight, and if you are dieting, you may get discouraged because of the bloating or weight gain. Typically this excess water disappears around the first day of the menstrual period.

ABDOMINAL CRAMPING:

> *Two weeks prior to menstruation I began to experience*
> *pain and swelling and exhaustion. By two days before*
> *menstruation I had cramping. And terrible cramps, nau-*
> *sea, and weakness came with the start of menstruation. I*
> *do not suffer from depression or mood swings.*
>
> *My abdomen feels tender, especially if I sit down fast.*
>
> *It's a feeling of a pull that goes from my vagina down*
> *both thighs.*

Premenstrual cramps, which sometimes feel a lot like menstrual cramps, can occur up to two weeks before the period begins. They may or may not be followed by heavy menstrual cramps. Often the cramping begins at midcycle, the time of ovulation, and either continues in full force or else abates until just before the period begins. Cramping may also be felt in the back, thighs, or vaginal area.

ACCIDENT-PRONENESS, LACK OF COORDINATION, SLURRED SPEECH:

> *I know I'm premenstrual when I start cutting my*
> *fingers slicing vegetables.*

One of the more subtle but troublesome symptoms of PMS is the decrease in physical coordination that can result in women tripping more easily, dropping things, feeling less able to carry out usually easy physical tasks. Some athletes and dancers say that their timing is off. Singers may find their voices altered, not as fine, and may dread performances premenstrually.

ACNE, HIVES, STYES, PIMPLE ERUPTIONS, RASHES:

> *When am I going to outgrow adolescence? I always*
> *have blackheads, but get a fresh crop of pimples monthly*
> *—and it takes nearly a month to get them to clear up.*

Acne is not *caused* by PMS, but many women, adult and teens, find that their acne become much worse premenstrually. Women who don't usually have skin problems may still break out with pimples or sores at this time of month. If a woman is prone to styes or other infections, including herpes, these problems may erupt premenstrually. Some women are more allergic to makeup; others report their makeup doesn't look right at this time of month.

ALCOHOL INTOLERANCE:

> *I became an alcoholic due to PMS because I found that*
> *if I lived like a zombie I wouldn't feel anything.*
>
> *My doctor told me a glass of wine might make me relax*
> *at night.*

Perhaps you don't usually notice any effects from four ounces of wine or a glass of beer, but premenstrually you may feel as though you'd had several times that amount. Furthermore, some women resort to alcohol as a solution to premenstrual mood changes and physical discomforts. There is therefore a clear-cut relationship between alcoholism and PMS. The combination of increased sensitivity and alcohol's depressing effect have resulted in a self-perpetuating pattern of alcohol consumption and depression.

ASTHMA: Asthma is certainly not caused by PMS, but there are women whose asthma occurs primarily premenstrually. This may or may not be in association with generalized increased infections and allergic reactions. Asthma is a condition that can be affected by infection, allergy, stress, and emotions.

BACK PAIN, JOINT PAIN, MUSCLE ACHES, STIFF NECK: Few people chart their aches and pains in relation to their menstrual cycles. Orthopedists are becoming increasingly aware, however, that unexplained recurrent back and other muscle pains may be related to a woman's cycle. Commonly the pains begin in one area, as with a stiff neck, and over the course of a week or so tend to travel to the back or legs. Traditionally these pains have simply been ignored as "women's complaints."

BREAST SWELLING AND PAIN:

> *I can't stand the sheet touching my breasts.*

> *The breast pain begins between one to two weeks before the onset of my period. The consistency of my breasts changes when the pain begins. They usually feel mildly lumpy, but premenstrually they become quite hard near my underarms and many small tube-shaped lumps can be felt around the outside of each breast. The lumps are very tender and hurt when touched. My breasts at this time feel extremely heavy and sore all over. Under my arms and on the part of my breasts closest to my underarms I feel extremely sharp pains. Sometimes I feel the pain all the way down my arm. The pain is usually greatest in the morning and at night. This breast pain lasts from one to two weeks before my period until two to three days after my period has started.*

The breast symptoms that occur with PMS can be mild or quite severe. The swelling and soreness can result in extreme sensitivity to any touch, including clothing. Breast cysts tend to become enlarged at this time, and women whose breast tissue is usually smooth may develop lumps. These symptoms usually disappear within a few days of the onset of the period.

CONFUSION, ABSENTMINDEDNESS, SPACINESS, INDECISIVENESS:

> *It's like a thin wall of glass is set up in my head.*

I've had some of my best moments in the courtroom even though I've felt premenstrually spacy inside. I can't explain it. I dread those days because of how I feel, but I always seem to come through. Sometimes I think I'm just going on automatic pilot.

Memory difficulties or a vague sense of "not thinking quite right" can occur premenstrually. Strangely, other people may have no idea that a woman is having this difficulty. These are intriguing symptoms because some extremely competent and highly functioning women report having them. They say that because of the pressure of their work they can overcome them. Unfortunately, others are severely incapacitated by these problems.

EATING DISORDERS, ANOREXIA, BULIMIA:

I know it seems like an exaggeration, but it's as though a hungry monster inside me were ready to devour anything sweet, especially chocolate. I'll stuff and stuff myself. Then after I'm done, I'm suddenly calm. I can't believe I lost control again. Sometimes I make myself throw up; sometimes I am just depressed and don't bother.

I have been a borderline anorexic for years. Premenstrually though, all I can think about is food. I stare at it, count calories in volume, imagine eating it. I rarely actually give in to bingeing, but it's hard not to.

We are living at a time when there is an epidemic of eating disorders among women. PMS greatly exacerbates these, partly because of the premenstrual cravings and changes in appetite. Women get into a pattern of binging premenstrually, followed by laxative use or self-induced vomiting, or by starvation between binges and after the period begins.

EYE DIFFICULTIES:

I can't read for fourteen days.

Regularly recurring problems can include excessive dryness of the eyes or tearing (to be differentiated from crying), difficulty focusing, and aching eyes.

FAINTING AND DIZZINESS: Sometimes in the absence of any diagnosed medical condition, women will experience these symptoms premenstrually.

FATIGUE, LETHARGY, TIREDNESS:

> *I think on those days that I'll never be able to move again. I mean, I really think that this is the end, that my body has quit on me.*

Women can experience fatigue throughout the premenstrual time or, more commonly, one or two days prior to the onset of menstruation. This pervasive sense of exhaustion can occur without any of the mood changes.

HAND TINGLING AND NUMBNESS: These can occur, only premenstrually, without any evidence of known neurological diseases that could account for them.

HEADACHES: All types of headaches, including migraines and tension headaches, can occur more frequently or solely during the premenstrual time for women with PMS. Often the migraines occur on the day before the period or during the first two days of bleeding. Some women have headaches starting shortly *after* their periods begin. This is not PMS, but it is a menstrually related phenomenon that is now being recognized because women have begun keeping track of when their headaches occur.

HEMORRHOIDS: Hemorrhoids are not caused by PMS, but they can be much more troublesome during that phase of the cycle. They tend to hurt more and they bleed more.

INFECTIONS: Many infections seem to occur on a regular basis premenstrually. These include sinus infections, sore throats, herpes (cold sores and genital herpes), skin boils, urinary tract infections, and others. These infections are caused by the usual organisms, but there seems to be a decrease in the body's resistance at this time and therefore an exacerbation of symptoms.

INSOMNIA: Premenstrual sleeplessness can occur independent of any mood changes and in women who otherwise sleep well. In fact, the insomnia often begins before other symptoms and may *contribute* to mood shifts, irritability, and depression. The insomnia can consist either of difficulty falling asleep at night or of awakening too early in the morning.

LACTATION DIFFICULTIES: Contrary to popular belief, women often menstruate while they are still nursing. Premenstrually they may find changes both in quality and quantity of the milk. Babies may react differently to nursing in the few days before menstruation. These changes are somewhat more frequent among women who are relactating or attempting to lactate in order to nurse an adopted baby.

MENSTRUAL CRAMPS (DYSMENORRHEA): These are *not* part of PMS. In fact, women with PMS more often have painless periods, though some do have both PMS and severe menstrual cramping. Women with PMS tend to look forward to getting their periods because of the relief they feel, even in the presence of cramps; women with dysmenorrhea more often dread their periods. The presence of menstrual cramps is *not* an indication of PMS.

NAUSEA: This occurs often in conjunction with dizziness and premenstrual cramping.

PALPITATIONS (HEART POUNDING), CARDIAC ARRHYTHMIAS (IRREGULAR HEARTBEATS):

> *I have anxious feelings with skin tingling, I have been hospitalized five times for heart palpitations. I've been to many doctors and they haven't found a cause for the heart palpitations.*

Cardiac irregularities can be an indication of serious and potentially dangerous cardiac conditions. Often, especially when they occur only premenstrually, a cause is not found, but they should always be thoroughly investigated.

SEIZURES:

> *My seizures come premenstrually even though they are treated with medication. I get scared and forget where I am and then I cry easily.*

Some women with seizure disorders find that their seizures are more common premenstrually. This is true of grand mal, petit mal, and temporal lobe seizures.

SENSITIVITY TO NOISE, TOUCH, SMELL:

> *Two weeks after my period, my breasts swell, joints ache, lower back pain. Then one week later, it's depression, sensitivity to loud noise, and general sense of loss of control.*

> *When I say to my mother, "That smells terrible," she says, "You must be getting your period."*

> *I don't want to be touched.*

> *I can't wear wool premenstrually.*

> *My jewelry begins to irritate me premenstrually.*

Women most often report an increased sensitivity to touch and hearing, but some also react strongly to certain smells. The sensitivity to sound ranges from being more bothered by a baby's crying to finding the radio or TV much too loud. The sensitivity to touch includes specific tender areas of the body as well as a generalized sensation of discomfort when the skin is touched.

SEX-DRIVE CHANGES:

> *One day of extreme fatigue every month—I could spend that day in bed. Despite extreme fatigue I experience hyper-sexuality, sexual thoughts, and a feeling of just barely keeping my sex drive under control.*

> *My husband and I have a good sex life, but premenstrually I couldn't care less and I know it hurts him to have me feel that way.*

These changes in sex drive will be described more fully in Chapter 17. Both increased and decreased libido can occur during the premenstrual phase of the cycle.

SWEET CRAVINGS, SALT CRAVINGS: The physiological changes in a woman's body premenstrually often result in hunger and specific food cravings. The most common foods craved are chocolate and salty chips. This is the time that is most difficult for dieting women because they find it hardest to refrain from sweets and often become discouraged because of their binges. As mentioned earlier, women caught in the cycle of anorexia, bingeing, and self-induced vomiting often have their most difficult times premenstrually. Liking chocolate per se is not a symptom of PMS, but driving out at midnight in a rainstorm to get it is indicative of having and giving into a strong craving. Doing this repeatedly shortly before you get your period is symptomatic of a premenstrual craving. If this behavior significantly interferes in your life, you have PMS.

URINARY DIFFICULTIES: Increased frequency of urination and burning on urination can occur premenstrually even in the absence of known infection. Some women seem to have an increase in the sensitivity of the urinary tract as well as of the vaginal areas.

WEIGHT GAIN: Some women feel as though they have gained weight even though the scale does not show an increase. Others have reported as much as a twelve-pound weight gain and loss monthly because of fluid retention. The weight gain of PMS is complicated by edema, food cravings, and binges.

Emotional Symptoms

ANGER, ANXIETY, CRYING, DEPRESSION, IRRITABILITY, LOSS OF SELF-ESTEEM, PANIC STATES, PARANOIA, SUICIDAL THOUGHTS, TENSION, VIOLENCE, WITHDRAWAL: The emotional symptoms, more than any others, most often bring women to seek help for PMS. In my first year of treating women with PMS, I was consulted by a woman who worked as a house cleaner in Nevada and had traveled to Boston at great financial hardship. When I asked her why she had come, she answered slowly, "Well, each month, my breasts hurt and my abdomen swells up . . ." She paused. I wondered at this answer because few women travel across the country for bloating and breast tenderness. "And," she continued, staring at the floor, "I'm a bitch."

She was describing PMS.

> *Just about a week before my periods I begin to go into a world of like a mental illness—crying jags, phobias about going outside, like impending doom—constantly thinking about dying. I am not a suicidal person, but I need help in this area.*
>
> *I become so snappish I have to keep myself from firing people on my staff.*
>
> *I feel as if I'm in a dark hole and can't get out.*

Obviously all these emotions are common to both men and women and can occur at all times of the month. It is their *cyclic* and often unexplained presence premenstrually that characterizes them as premenstrual syndrome.

Women frequently seek help for their PMS because of the emotional costs and pain to their families, friends, and co-workers. They are often more worried about the effects of their PMS on others than on themselves. Women with children frequently seek help because they fear losing control around the children or hurting them as a result of their unpredictable mood changes.

> *I have a feeling of hatred toward others, and I withdraw so I won't hurt anyone.*

Some women experience what feels to them like a complete personality change, as though an outside force had just replaced Dr. Jekyll with Mr. Hyde. This change often includes feelings of anger, loss of control, and despair, much of which disappears with the onset of menstruation. The woman is left with a memory of having "been someone other than her present self," and with guilt for emotions expressed and actions taken during that time.

I'd even be okay if I knew I'd always be premenstrual.
Even while I'm angry with my husband I know I will
change and regret what I am saying. If I could be angry
consistently I'd be better. It's the change that's so difficult.

The change is unpredictable and often takes place without warning. It can be a matter of waking up one morning feeling tense, angry, irritable, knowing that anything anyone says will seem wrong, that anything which doesn't go as planned will result in anger or tears beyond what the reality of the situation would warrant. An attorney who premenstrually is experiencing sadness might lose a case and then believe that to be the cause of her sadness, when on another day the same loss would be taken in stride. If she is feeling angry and someone says something that annoys her, a woman may react out of proportion and even assume that what was said or done is the cause of her feeling. People around her are often left feeling that they can't do anything right.

I know I'm premenstrual when I'm driving along and
suddenly I find myself calling other drivers assholes! I
never use that word at any other time.

Some mornings I just feel this terrible anger in me. I'm
climbing the walls and I think I pick a fight with my
husband just for the release of the tension. I tell myself I
have reason to be angry at the time, but I know inside I'm
needing to fight with him.

For many women, however, the personality change is not so complete, nor are the issues so unrelated to reality as they would like to believe. Our society discourages the expression of anger by women, and during the premenstrual period those feelings may be less easily held in check. Many women have said that this is the one time when they can say whatever is on their minds.

Often the issues over which a woman is upset premenstrually are real ones, but at this time she is unable to express them constructively. Once the "loss of control" has passed, the woman, filled with guilt for how she expressed herself, looks back and says, "Oh, it really isn't important. I was just premenstrual." Those around her tend also to dismiss her complaints with "Oh, she was just being premenstrual." The validity of her concerns is thus denied both by the woman and by others. She feels guilty for her reaction, brushes it off, and like the perpetual dieter, promises herself that it won't happen again.

> *As I began to understand my PMS I saw that I had been like a pot with a heavy lid. When I wasn't premenstrual and something was on my mind, I just stuck it in the pot and forgot about it. But then when I was premenstrual it was as though the lid was loosened and all the stuff I'd been burying came blasting out at everyone, including me.*

Being in Control

For many women, being in control at all times is basic to their functioning and sense of stability. Physiological changes that lessen control of their emotions can threaten their self-esteem, identity, and sense of femininity. Few women actually lose control, but the feeling that it is about to be lost can be terrifying.

Women tend to be defensive about their premenstrual experiences. One woman described her despair about PMS like this: "I'm a graphic artist, but for two weeks out of the month I'm worthless at work. I just can't do as well as I can the rest of the time." Asked about her general performance, whether she thought she contributed as much to her job as the men in her office, she quickly and easily responded, "Oh yes, I'm certainly as good as they are. I'm actually the best person in the department." Asked if sometimes the men perform at less than their full potential, she said, "Sure, every time something goes wrong at home or in business, they're useless at work too. It happens to them all the time." Women often hold themselves to a standard of performance that on a sustained basis is unrealistic for anyone.

Heightened Consciousness

PMS in some ways resembles an altered state of consciousness, an experience of being in a different world, of looking at life through a magnifying lens. It is often a world with its own internal consistency. Some women describe an enhancement of creativity and perceptiveness, a richness of sensation and imagery lacking at other times.

A sculptor described her special abilities when she was premenstrual.

> *There is a quality to my work and to my vision which just isn't there the rest of the month. I look forward to being premenstrual for its effect on my creativity, although some of the other symptoms create strains with my family.*

Another woman, prone to depression, described the journal she kept:

> *When I am premenstrual I can write with such clarity and depth that after I get my period I don't recognize that those were my thoughts or that I could have written anything so profound.*

An aide in a nursing home became upset about the treatment of the patients when she was premenstrual. When she saw the old people neglected and suffering, she often broke down in tears and harbored fantasies of calling the health department to close the place. When she was not premenstrual, she still did not like what she saw, but she would become more "realistic" and able to cope with the situation.

CHAPTER 4

❖

Causes of PMS

A WOMAN WITH PMS is basically healthy, and some of the problem in recognizing PMS is that each system seems to work well *part of each month.* Most of the time the woman's body knows how to excrete water and salt efficiently. Women with PMS do not walk around with massive edema all month, like people with various other disorders. They are not in a rage all the time, as are some men and women who are generally considered disturbed. As for basic reproductive functioning, women with PMS usually do ovulate, do conceive, and do carry to term.

PMS does represent a physiological problem, but it is in the regulatory mechanism of the body's functioning. Signals are crossed, lost, or distorted, but only some of the time. It is as though the body were an orchestra. Each instrument or set of instruments is able to play well, but then *part of the month* something goes wrong with the conductor.

To believe that a regulatory process is not working correctly is different from believing that many individual parts of your body are breaking down. To say, "I have a generally healthy body, but there is something wrong in the balance or homeostasis for part of the month," is quite different from "My body is falling apart."

Where Is the Conductor?

As far as is understood, the regulatory center of the body resides in the hypothalamus, an area in the center of the brain where the neurological and endocrine systems are integrated. This area receives nerve and hormonal input from the other parts of the brain and from the rest of the body; then it sends out messages controlling the nervous and endocrine functions of the body. It seems likely therefore that the hypothalamus is the conductor that in PMS goes awry during part of each menstrual cycle.

The hypothalamus is involved, either directly or indirectly, in the following bodily processes:

- It secretes hormones and stimulates the anterior pituitary gland. This gland in turn affects the following:
  · breasts—stimulation of milk production directly and breast tissue fullness indirectly.
  · thyroid gland—controls basic metabolic functioning of cells.
  · adrenal glands—results in steroid production and partial blood glucose control.
  · ovaries—hormones from pituitary gland stimulate development of cells that lead to ovulation and to estrogen and progesterone production. These hormones also affect libido.
  · tissue and bone growth through the secretion of growth hormone.
- It stimulates the posterior pituitary gland, whose hormones affect uterine contractions and labor as well as water and electrolyte balance.
- It directly stimulates portions of the autonomic nervous system, thereby affecting
  · heart rate.
  · blood pressure.
  · heat regulation through shivering, panting, sweating.
  · gastrointestinal movement and glucose level regulation.
  · constriction and relaxation of bronchial tubes in the lungs.

Specific centers within the hypothalamus also regulate more specific functions, many of which seem to operate poorly premenstrually.

- A thermoregulatory center adjusts the body to maintain body temperatures.

- An appetite center registers both hunger and satisfaction, thus influencing eating behavior.
- A weight control center seems to "set" body weight.
- Specific emotional centers in the hypothalamus are poorly understood, but animal studies have demonstrated the following:
  · stimulation of some centers produces responses suggestive of reward and punishment.
  · stimulation of punishment centers results in a pattern of behavior called rage because the animal responds as if to attack.
  · stimulation of some areas causes reactions that seem to be anxiety and fear.
- Susceptibility to rage seems to follow destruction of some parts of the hypothalamus in humans.

When you look at the long list of PMS symptoms in the previous chapter, you can see how many of them can be seen as being related to hypothalamic functioning.

What Affects the Hypothalamus?

1. The hypothalamus operates by *feedback*—i.e., by responding to what is already happening in the body. If the temperature is too high or too low it directs the appropriate changes in activity, sweating or shivering, to bring the temperature back within normal range. This kind of subtle shifting is occurring all the time in response to physical conditions as well as to levels of circulating hormones. Too much is a signal to produce less, and vice versa.

2. The hypothalamus responds to *neurotransmitters,* chemicals secreted by nerve endings. These substances have been related to mood changes. The hypothalamus is bathed in neurotransmitters, which in turn stimulate hypothalamic activity and hormone production or even become transformed into hormones themselves. This mechanism is important because it explains how stress and mood can *themselves* result in hormonal changes.

3. The hypothalamus produces more or less of some hormones depending on the amount of light the body is exposed to. It is sensitive to day/night cycles as well as to monthly ones.

4. The hypothalamus is directly connected to other parts of the brain and receives stimulation from them. For instance, certain nerve fibers connect olfactory (smell) centers with the hypothalamus, so stimulation by smell can affect the hypothalamus.

5. While less is known about these factors, it is likely that the hypothalamus, like other areas of the body, is also affected by heredity, trauma, nutrition (including hormones ingested in foods) infection, and unexplained individual idiosyncrasies.

None of this explains why the hypothalamus does not function well for part of the month. In fact, no one knows that. Nevertheless, pieces of the puzzle are beginning to be understood, most of them related to parts of individual systems affected. To return to the analogy of the orchestra, we are beginning to find what is wrong with some of the players premenstrually as well as to understand more about what influences the conductor.

The following are some of the proposed explanations of PMS:

progesterone deficiency and estrogen
   excess
prostaglandin deficiency
vitamin deficiency
magnesium deficiency
hypoglycemia
allergy to one's own hormones

fluid retention
prolactin (pituitary hormone) excess
stress
endorphin (brain opiates) deficiency or
   abnormality
emotional illness

None of these theories have been proven, however. They are what is known as working hypotheses, theories that bear looking into as possible causes and that lend themselves to future testing and experimentation.

What Does Not Cause PMS

There are no good cross-cultural studies of PMS, studies comparing this condition in widely different societies; nor is much known about it historically. Most of what has been written about the cycle has been about menstruation itself rather than about PMS. And much of this literature has been clouded by the stigma attached to menstruation.

Because PMS is so elusive and confusing, there is a tendency both for women and their doctors to assign blame to whatever is seen as a defect. Obese women often believe that if they lost weight their PMS would get better. This unfortunately is not the case: PMS affects women of all sizes and weights.

Women home with children often assume that if they had jobs outside their home, their PMS would improve, while women with careers have said, "I envy women at home because they don't have to function on a job. They have it easier." The reality is that women at home with or without children have PMS; women with careers, even very successful careers, have PMS. There may be other reasons for getting or giving up jobs, but curing PMS isn't one of them. PMS is not caused by housework, children, or professions.

Mental illness does not cause PMS. Women can be emotionally disturbed with or without PMS. These disturbances occur regardless of the menstrual period. And women who are emotionally healthy, aware of feelings, and able to cope well can still have severe PMS. There is no evidence that PMS is more or less common among women who have emotional disturbances, but PMS can be more devastating to women whose sense of identity and control are already precarious.

Perfectionism and PMS do seem to be related. Women who maintain exceptionally high standards of behavior and control appear to be more easily shaken by finding themselves periodically unable to meet those standards. PMS is probably not more common in these women, but they often have a more difficult time dealing with it.

PMS is not caused by other people. It may be worse in stressful situations and in dysfunctioning relationships, but PMS resides within the individual woman who experiences the symptoms.

CHAPTER 5

Premenstrual Magnification (PMM)

I have been a diabetic for twelve years and take insulin shots twice a day. Premenstrually my diabetes gets out of control and I have much more trouble keeping my sugar levels down.

Why another label, another "sickness"?

Because too many women with *premenstrual magnification* of their symptoms are being told that they do not have a cyclic disturbance related to their menstrual periods. Women are being turned away from PMS clinics because they don't have a symptom-free week each month. They are being told that they are suggestible women imagining that they have PMS or trying to have it. The danger in giving a name to still another condition related to the menstrual cycle is that another female experience is thereby being labeled an illness. However, I believe there is a greater danger in denial of some women's experiences.

Women with premenstrual magnification, or PMM, unlike those with PMS, are to some extent ill throughout the entire month, but they are *worse* premenstrually. Whether they suffer from asthma, epilepsy, diabetes, depression, arthritis, or almost any other disease, their difficulties are increased premenstrually and are then partially relieved with the onset of menstruation. Unlike women with PMS, when these women get their periods they do not have the dramatic relief from all their symptoms because the underlying disorder is still there.

PMM, like PMS, can be mild and barely noticeable or severe and incapacitating. The magnification can be one of joy, excitement, or creativity too. And you can have *both* PMM and PMS. Your headaches may be present all month but worse premenstrually, while your bloating and depression may occur only premenstrually. Or you may be agoraphobic all month, although more severely so before your period, but have breast pain, cramps, and outbursts of anger *only* premenstrually.

PMM doesn't appear to fit classical definitions of PMS because some symptoms are present all month, but the cyclicity is the same in that symptoms are heightened or magnified during the time between ovulation and menstruation. Only the presence of a constant underlying disease marks the difference between the two. The chart on page 48 illustrates this pattern of symptoms.

> *In a good month I'm usually very tired ten days before I start bleeding. I wake up tired and go to bed tired. In a bad month I'm tired almost every day. I will sleep an hour at lunch and then anywhere from one to two hours when I get home from work. I've been mildly depressed as long as I can remember.*

Treatment of PMM is not always the same as for PMS. Many times the underlying disorder must be treated first, as if PMS were not also present. For instance, treating depression tends only to remove the underlying depression but still leaves a sometimes severe premenstrual fluctuation of mood. So along with, or after trying to alleviate the constant depression, treatment for the PMS may also become necessary.

Women with PMM often describe feeling different premenstrually, even though their symptoms are present all month.

> *I know I'm depressed other times, but it* feels *different premenstrually. It takes on a characteristic of doom, impending doom.*

Although it might seem to an observer or health care practitioner that a woman is ill all the time, she may feel her illness more acutely premenstrually.

My asthma is usually set off by colds, so I am always susceptible to attacks. I have realized that the ones that send me to the emergency room seem to occur the day before my period starts. Sometimes I even begin to menstruate while I am still in the ER.

Two years ago I was diagnosed as having lupus. Premenstrually it usually gives me more problems, especially with my skin rashes. My joints ache more, too.

Women with PMM need to know they are not isolated cases of a rare disorder but rather that they share a common experience. The lesson of PMM is in listening to women about what they are *feeling.* Then when their symptoms don't seem to make sense or fit into previous beliefs about a disease, the challenge is to question the beliefs, not the women.

CHAPTER 6

⊠

Diagnosis

Do I/Does She Have PMS?

There is no mystery to the diagnosis of PMS. In fact it is most easily made on the basis of the "Aha!" experience. If you read stories about women with PMS and say to yourself, "That's me," then you probably have PMS. If you react to the same stories and descriptions with "How could anyone feel/be that way?" then you probably don't.

There are currently no reliable chemical, physical, or psychological tests to determine PMS. There is charting, which a woman does herself, and there are several diagnostic criteria that are suggestive of PMS, although not by any means diagnostic. Even charting can be difficult to evaluate because there are women who may have some symptoms all month long but who still insist that "it feels different" premenstrually. Also, charting is limited because it describes experiences only in words or symbols and therefore cannot be used to validate their authenticity. PMS is an experience that a woman either has or doesn't have. The only absolute criteria is the presence of the symptoms in the *premenstrual phase* of her cycle and their dramatic alleviation close to the onset of her menses.

Common Characteristics of PMS

While the "many symptoms of PMS" include some that are common and some that are rare, the following collection of characteristics are almost always present among women with PMS. In some treatment centers, they are actually considered diagnostic of the syndrome, but my experience shows that at times they may not all be present.

1. Onset following puberty, pregnancy, extreme weight loss with temporary cessation of periods, use of birth control pills, tubal ligation, ovarian surgery, or hysterectomy.

2. Made worse by pregnancy (it can be increasingly severe with subsequent pregnancies), cessation of periods from weight loss, birth control pills, tubal ligation, ovarian surgery, hysterectomy.

3. Miscarriage and toxemia of pregnancy seem to be more common among women with PMS.

4. Postpartum depression may be the beginning of PMS and occurs more frequently among women who have had PMS. As menstruation resumes after delivery, the depression may change from a constant one to a depression cyclicly related to the period.

5. Pregnancy is usually a positive experience for women with PMS, especially after the first trimester. Often they describe being pregnant as the one time they feel "wonderful." This characteristic is ironic because women have at times become pregnant as a solution to depression only to discover that their PMS is worse after they give birth.

6. Menstruation is more often painless. There is no particular cycle length or type of menstrual bleeding characteristic of PMS. Cycles may be long, short, or irregular; bleeding may be light or heavy, with or without clots.

7. The history of side effects on birth control pills for women with PMS usually includes headache, weight gain, and depression. Often the symptoms warrant discontinuation of the pills.

8. Acute symptoms (migraines headaches, panic attacks, epilepsy, depression, etc.) often follow long gaps between meals—i.e., five hours in

the day or thirteen hours overnight. In this way, many of the manifestations of PMS resemble hypoglycemia, a condition in which the blood sugar drops either too low or too quickly. In PMS these symptoms occur premenstrually.

9. As indicated earlier, food cravings and binges can be quite severe for women with PMS. For women with mild difficulties the response may be "I always know when my period is due because I find myself eyeing chocolate and touching potato-chip bags in the grocery store." In severe cases women may eat entire cakes or half gallons of ice cream in one sitting. Eating disorders are most difficult to control at this time because self-control is at its lowest. For women who are dieting, this is a most difficult time because they tend to binge and then hate themselves for failing at their diet; then they try to fast, which may bring on hypoglycemic symptoms.

10. Women can be much more sensitive to alcohol premenstrually. In addition some women turn to alcohol for relief of their tension. Combined with their increased sensitivity and with alcohol's depressive effect, this may lead to more drinking and depression. Furthermore, certain women who have repeatedly turned to alcohol for relief of PMS symptoms have become alcoholics.

11. Sex-drive changes premenstrually can take the form of either an increase or decrease in sexual desire. Some women lose any desire for sex premenstrually while others have an increase, especially in the few days just before their periods (see Chapter 17).

12. Women with PMS typically experience a sense of *relief* when they get their periods. This relief is usually abrupt, occurring between twelve hours prior to bleeding to twenty-four hours after the period begins. Even when the menses itself is painful or exhausting, women usually say they feel much better as soon as they bleed.

Charting PMS Symptoms

Charting symptoms is an important key to diagnosis, since it provides a picture of when the symptoms are occurring in relation to the menses, which symptoms are related to the cycle, and which are present at other times too. Approach charting with a sense of curiosity and exploration rather than a desire to prove or disprove whether you have PMS. Invariably women find that some of what they thought was PMS also occurs at other times and that other symptoms thought to be irrelevant actually occur premenstrually. The charting of symptoms is a fairly recent technique that may help us discover new relationships between the menstrual cycle and health or illness.

Remember, charting should not be oppressive, but for women who want to know precisely when and which symptoms may be related to PMS, keeping track is one of the best ways to get that information. And remember that charting is just a record of *experience.*

STEP-BY-STEP CHARTING: Charting itself can be simple or complicated depending on what is being recorded and how much energy you have to devote to the task. The simplest form is like Chart 1 that follows. As a practical matter, the chart has 8 columns instead of 12 to give you more room to mark symptoms. A wall calendar or small yearly calendar can also be useful. What is important is to be able to see graphically when symptoms are occurring in relation to the menstrual cycle. For instance, a daily plan book works less well because the time relationships are harder to see.

In Chart 1, the numbers along the left margin represent the days of the month. Mark the individual months across the top. Note the dates of your menstrual period with an M. If you have spotting for a day or two before or after your period, mark those days with an S.

CHART I

SYMPTOMS   INITIALS

1. _____ _____

2. _____ _____   Menstruation: $\textcircled{M}$

3. _____ _____   Date charting began: _____

MONTHS

1								
2								
3								
4								
5								
6								
7								
8								
9								
10								
11								
12								
13								
14								
15								
16								
17								
18								
19								
20								
21								
22								
23								
24								
25								
26								
27								
28								
29								
30								
31								

CHART 2

If your period was from January 15 through 20, February 14 through 18, and March 17 through 21, your chart will look like Chart 2. Although the average menstrual cycle length is twenty-eight days, it varies considerably from woman to woman, and the length may also change at different times in a particular woman's life. Cycle length is not related to PMS, nor is cycle regularity, nor is the number of days of bleeding. Traditionally the days of the cycle are numbered beginning with the first day of bleeding of one menstrual period and ending with the first day of bleeding of the next period.

Note that here the cycle beginning January 15 was thirty days, the next one thirty-one days.

CHART 2

SYMPTOMS   INITIALS

1. _____   _____

2. _____   _____   Menstruation: (M)

3. _____   _____   Date charting began: _____

MONTHS

	January		February		March									
1				(18)		(16)							
2				(19)		(17)							
3				(20)		(18)							
4				(21)		(19)							
5				(22)		(20)							
6				(23)		(21)							
7				(24)		(22)							
8				(25)		(23)							
9				(26)		(24)							
10				(27)		(25)							
11				(28)		(26)							
12				(29)		(27)							
13				(30)		(28)							
14			(M)	(1)		(29)							
15	(M)	(1)	(M)	(2)		(30)							
16	(M)	(2)	(M)	(3)		(31)							
17	(M)	(3)	(M)	(4)	(M)	(1)							
18	(M)	(4)	(M)	(5)	(M)	(2)							
19	(M)	(5)		(6)	(M)	(3)							
20	(M)	(6)		(7)	(M)	(4)							
21		(7)		(8)	(M)	(5)							
22		(8)		(9)		(6)							
23		(9)		(10)		(7)							
24		(10)		(11)		(8)							
25		(11)		(12)		(9)							
26		(12)		(13)		(10)							
27		(13)		(14)		(11)							
28		(14)		(15)		(12)							
29		(15)	✕			(13)							
30		(16)	✕			(14)							
31		(17)				(15)							

CHART 3

If you also had breast tenderness, which you represent with a B, from January 4 through 15, February 10 through 14, and March 5 through 15, your chart would look like Chart 3.

CHART 3

SYMPTOMS   INITIALS

1. _Breast Tenderness_ _____   __B__

2. _____ _____   Menstruation: (M)

3. _____ _____   Date charting began: _____

MONTHS

	January	February	March						
1									
2									
3									
4	B								
5	B		B						
6	B		B						
7	B		B						
8	B		B						
9	B		B						
10	B	B	B						
11	B	B	B						
12	B	B	B						
13	B	B	B						
14	B	(M) B	B						
15	(M) B	(M)	B						
16	(M)	(M)	(M)						
17	(M)	(M)	(M)						
18	(M)	(M)	(M)						
19	(M)		(M)						
20	(M)								
21									
22									
23									
24									
25									
26									
27									
28									
29		✕							
30		✕							
31		✕							

CHART 4

Chart 4 shows clearly that this woman's symptoms are occurring each month prior to the onset of her period and that her tension is relieved when the period begins. It also indicates that May was an easier month, with only three days of tension. It is common for premenstrual symptoms to vary as to length, intensity, and type.

CHART 4

SYMPTOMS   INITIALS

1. _Tension_____   _T_

2. _____ _____   Menstruation: (M)

3. _____ _____   Date charting began: _____

MONTHS

	January	February	March	April	May	June		
1								
2								
3						T		
4						T		
5			T			T		
6			T			T		
7		T	T			T		
8		T	T			T		
9	T	T	T			T		
10	T	T		T		T		
11	T	T	T	T	T	(M)		
12	T	T	T	T	T	(M)		
13	T	T	T	T	T	(M)		
14	T	T	T	T	(m)	(M)		
15	T	T	T	T	(M)			
16	T	T	(M)		(M)			
17	T	(M)	(M)	T	(M)			
18	(M)	(M)	(M)	T				
19	(M)	(M)	(M)					
20	(M)	(M)		T				
21	(M)			T				
22	(M)			T				
23				(m)				
24				(m)				
25				(m)				
26				(M)				
27				(M)				
28								
29		X						
30		X						
31		X		X		X		

CHART 5

Three symptoms appear in Chart 5: breast tenderness, lethargy, and depression. Notice that the breast changes often precede the emotional ones, although this is not always true. The lethargy tended to begin about a week before and to last through one or two days of the period. The depression lifted with the onset of menstruation. Note also that in one month there were no breast symptoms at all.

CHART 5

SYMPTOMS   INITIALS

1. Breast Tenderness _____   B

2. Lethargy _____   L   Menstruation: (M)

3. Depression _____   D   Date charting began: _____

MONTHS

	January	February	March	April	May	June	July	August
1		B		B		B L D		
2	B	B		B	D	B L D		
3	B	B D	B D	B D	L D	B L D		
4	B	B D	B D	B D	L D	B L D		
5	B D	B L D	B D	B L D	L D	B L D		
6	B D	B L D	B D	B L D	L D	B L D		
7	B D	B L D	B L D	B L D	(M) L D	(M) L		
8	B D	B L D	B L D	B L D	(M) L	(M)		
9	B L D	B L D	B L D	B L D	(M)	(M)		
10	B L D	B L D	B L D	B L D	(M)	(M)		
11	B L D	B L D	B L D	B L D	(M)	(M)		
12	B L D	(M) L	B L D	B L D		(M)		
13	B L D	(M)	(M) L	(M) L				
14	B L D	(M)	(M)	(M)				
15	B L D	(M)	(M)	(M)				
16	(M) L		(M)	(M)				
17	(M) L		(M)					
18	(M)		(M)					
19	(M)		(M)					
20								
21								
22								
23								
24								
25								
26								
27					B			
28					B			
29		✕			B			
30		✕	B	✕	B L D			
31	B	✕	B	✕	B L D	✕		

CHART 6

On Chart 6, the bloating clearly occurs only premenstrually, but you will notice that the anger has occurred at other times. There are two possible explanations. One is that further charting will show that the anger is predominantly premenstrual; the other that there are other reasons she is experiencing and expressing anger. Where there is anger at other times of the month, women often say that the premenstrual anger and depression "feels different."

CHART 6

SYMPTOMS   INITIALS

1. Anger — A
2. Depression — D
3. Bloating — B

Menstruation: (M)

Date charting began: _____

MONTHS

	January	February	March	April	May	June	July	August
1	(M)	(M)	(M)	(M)	B D	(M)	(m)	
2	(M)	(M)	(M)	(M)	(M)	(M)	(m)	
3	(M)	(M)	(M)	(M)	(M)	(M)	(M)	
4	(M)		(M)	(M) A	(M)	(M)		
5				A	(M)			
6						A		
7						A		
8								
9								
10		A						
11		A						
12		A						
13								
14								
15								
16						A		
17				B		D A		
18				B		B D A		
19				B		B D		
20	D	B D		B		B D		
21	B D	B D				B D		
22	B D	B D		B D	A	B D		
23	B D	B D		B D	A	B		
24	B D	B D A	B	B D A	B A	B D		
25	B D A	B D A	B	B D A	B A	B D		
26	B D A	B A	B D A	B D A	B D	B		
27	B D A	B A	B D A	B D A	B D	B D		
28	B D A	B A	B D A	B D	B D	(M)		
29	B D A	✕	B D A	B D	B D	(M)		
30	(M)	✕	B D A	B D	B D	(M)		
31	(M)	✕	(M)	✕	B D	✕		

CHART 7

Another way of charting symptoms is by severity. When it isn't clear that
a symptom occurs *only* premenstrually, you can chart its intensity on a
scale. Instead of recording three different symptoms, a woman who is
usually anxious rates the *level* of anxiety on a scale in which 1 = mild,
2 = moderate, and 3 = severe. In this way she is able to chart the
relationship between the severity of her symptoms and her menstrual
cycle. Clearly, although she has anxiety much of the month, it is more
severe premenstrually. This is an example of PMM, premenstrual magnification.

CHART 7

SYMPTOMS   INITIALS

1. *Mild* — *1*
2. *Moderate* — *2*
3. *Severe* — *3*

Menstruation: (M)
Date charting began: _____

MONTHS   *Anxiety*

	January	February	March	April	May	June	July	August
1			(M)	(M) 1	(M) 3	(M) 1		
2			(M)	(M) 1	(M) 1	(M)		
3		1	(M) 1	3	(M) 1	(M)		
4		1	(M) 1	1	(M) 1	(M)		
5		1	(M) 1	1	(M)			
6		2	1	1				
7		2	2	1	1			
8		1	2	2	1			
9		1	1					
10			1					
11			1					
12		1		1				
13		1		2				
14		1	3	1				
15		2	3	1				
16			1					
17			1	3				
18	3	1	1	3				
19	3	1	3	3				
20	3	3	3	3				
21	3	3	3	2				
22	3	3	2	2				
23	3	3	3	1				
24	2	3	3	2				
25	3	1	3	3	3			
26	2	3	2	3	3			
27	3	1	2	3	3			
28	(M)	(M)	3	3	3			
29	(M)		(M) 3	3	3			
30	(M) 1		(M) 3	3	3			
31	(M) 1		(M) 1		(M)			

CHART 8

Sometimes there are so many symptoms and so little clarity as to which ones are related to the cycle that the charting has to be expanded. One way is to use each chart for a separate month. Insert the *symptoms* across the top of the chart, and in the columns either use check marks for the presence of a symptom or use the scale of 1 to 3 to describe severity of symptoms. Charts 8, 9, and 10 represent three months of charting of multiple symptoms.

In January it is clear that this woman's anxiety is premenstrual. Her insomnia begins premenstrually but *continues,* so only further charting will show if there is a pattern. The rage occurred three times, twice premenstrually, so this requires more charting. Headaches seem to be scattered throughout the month. She also had what she described as "weird feelings" that she thought were only premenstrual. They consisted of a slight dizziness, disorientation, and difficulty focusing. Colors seemed sharper and her body felt slightly "strange." In January these feelings indeed occurred only premenstrually. Sinus difficulties, which she had thought to be related to her period on charting, seemed to come *after* her period began and to last into the first week postmenstrually. In January she also had a few days of nausea and marked this on the chart under "other."

CHART 8

SYMPTOMS   INITIALS

1. _____ _____

2. _____ _____   Menstruation: (M)

3. _____ _____   Date charting began: _____

~~MONTHS~~ SYMPTOMS   JANUARY

Other:

	Menstruation	Anxiety	Insomnia	Rage	Headaches	Weird Feelings	Sinus	
1				✓	✓			
2					✓			
3					✓			
4					✓			
5					✓			
6								
7								
8								
9								
10								
11		✓						n
12		✓						a
13		✓		✓				u
14		✓		✓		✓		s
15		✓	✓			✓		e
16		✓	✓			✓		a
17	(M)		✓			✓		
18	(M)		✓					
19	(M)		✓				✓	
20	(M)		✓				✓	
21	(M)		✓		✓		✓	
22			✓		✓		✓	
23			✓		✓		✓	
24					✓		✓	
25					✓			
26					✓			
27								
28					✓			
29					✓			
30								
31								

CHART 9

The February chart shows a similar pattern, with the anxiety, rage, and weird feelings clearly premenstrual. The insomnia does not seem to be related to this woman's cycle, and sinus problems again follow the menses.

CHART 9

SYMPTOMS   INITIALS

1. _____ _____

2. _____ _____   Menstruation: (M)

3. _____ _____   Date charting began: _____

~~MONTHS~~ SYMPTOMS   FEBRUARY

Other:

	Menstruation	Anxiety	Insomnia	Rage	Headaches	Weird Feelings	Sinus	
1								
2								
3			✓		✓			
4			✓		✓			
5								
6								
7								
8								
9								nausea
10		✓			✓	✓		
11		✓			✓	✓		
12		✓				✓		
13		✓		✓		✓		
14		✓		✓		✓		
15	(M)			✓		✓		
16	(M)			✓		✓		
17	(M)				✓			
18	(M)				✓		✓	
19					✓		✓	
20					✓		✓	
21					✓		✓	
22			✓		✓		✓	
23			✓		✓			
24			✓					
25			✓					
26			✓					
27								
28								
29								
30								
31								

CHART 10

By the third month (Chart 10) the pattern is even clearer. If you look back over the previous cycles, it is clear that the anxiety, rage, and "weird feelings" are premenstrual. Insomnia and headaches seem to occur at any time in the cycle. The nausea was premenstrual for two months but then did not recur, so it is unclear whether it is cycle-related. One episode of bingeing occurred premenstrually in March, and although this is probably cycle-related, that cannot really be determined without more charting.

CHART 10

SYMPTOMS   INITIALS

1. _____   _____

2. _____   _____   Menstruation: (M)

3. _____   _____   Date charting began: _____

~~MONTHS~~ SYMPTOMS   MARCH

Other:

	Menstruation	Anxiety	Insomnia	Rage	Headaches	Weird Feelings	Sinus	
1								
2		✓			✓			
3					✓			
4					✓			
5		✓						
6								
7								
8		✓						
9								
10								
11					✓			
12					✓			
13		✓			✓	✓		
14		✓	✓	✓		✓		*Bingeing
15		✓	✓	✓		✓		
16	(M)	✓	✓	✓				
17	(M)							
18	(M)		✓					
19	(M)		✓					
20			✓				✓	
21			✓				✓	
22			✓				✓	
23			✓				✓	
24			✓				✓	
25			✓				✓	
26								
27								
28								
29								
30								
31								

CHART 11

Sometimes the symptoms shift in severity during the premenstrual phase. They usually begin at the time of ovulation. They may then get better for a few days and then become severe again, or they may remain constant. In Chart 11, the irritability around the 22 and 23 of each month represents a symptom related to the time of ovulation.

CHART II

SYMPTOMS   INITIALS

1. Irritability   I
2. Bloating   B
3. Depression   D

Menstruation: (M)

Date charting began: _____

MONTHS

	January	February	March	April						
1		I		D						
2		I		D						
3				D I						
4				D I						
5				D						
6			I D							
7	(M)		I D	(M)						
8	(M)		(M)	(M)						
9	(M)		(M)	(M)						
10	(M)	(M)	(M)	(M)						
11		(M)	(M)							
12		(M)	(M)							
13		(M)								
14										
15										
16										
17										
18										
19										
20										
21			I							
22	I		I D							
23	I D	I								
24	I	I								
25		I								
26		I								
27										
28	I									
29	I	X								
30	I		D	X						
31		X	D							

CHART 12

Another way to chart symptoms is simply to use S to represent the presence of symptoms. In chart 12 the pattern is one of premenstrual difficulties every other month. Symptoms can occur regularly every other month, every third or fourth month, or irregularly. Some women have a cycle in which each month is more severe than the previous month for four or five months. Then an easy month occurs, followed by increasing symptoms again.

CHART 12

SYMPTOMS   INITIALS

1. _Symptoms_____   _S_

2. _____   _____   Menstruation: Ⓜ

3. _____   _____   Date charting began: _____

MONTHS

	June	July	August	September	October	November	December	January
1								
2					S			
3								
4							S	
5							S	
6					S		S	
7			S		S		S	
8			S		S		S	
9	S		S		S		S	
10	S		S				S	
11	S		S				S	
12	S		S		S	Ⓜ		
13	S		S	Ⓜ	S	Ⓜ	Ⓜ	
14	S		S	Ⓜ	Ⓜ	Ⓜ	Ⓜ	
15	S		Ⓜ	Ⓜ	Ⓜ	Ⓜ	Ⓜ	
16	S		Ⓜ	Ⓜ	Ⓜ		Ⓜ	
17	S	Ⓜ	Ⓜ	Ⓜ	Ⓜ		Ⓜ	
18	Ⓜ	Ⓜ	Ⓜ		Ⓜ			
19	Ⓜ	Ⓜ						
20	Ⓜ	Ⓜ						
21	Ⓜ							
22								
23								
24								
25								
26								
27								
28								
29								
30								
31	✕			✕		✕		

CHART 13

Symptoms can be so severe that they spread into the good weeks. When outbursts disrupt family and work, little peaceful or balanced time may be left. What is important then is to separate out the symptoms to gain an understanding of what is directly related to PMS and what is aftermath.

CHART 13

SYMPTOMS   INITIALS

1. _Symptoms_____   __S__

2. _____   _____   Menstruation: (M)

3. _____   _____   Date charting began: _____

MONTHS

	January	February	March	April				
1		S	S	S				
2		S	S	S				
3		S	S	S				
4		S	S	S				
5		S	S	S				
6		S	S	S				
7		S	S	S				
8		S	S	S				
9		S	S	S				
10		S	S	S				
11		S	S	S				
12		S	S	S				
13		S	S	S				
14		S	S	(M) S				
15		(M) S	(M) S	(M) S				
16		(M) S	(m) S	(m) S				
17		(M) S	(M) S	(M)				
18	(M)	(M) S	(M) S					
19	(M)	(M)						
20	(M)							
21	(M)							
22	(M)		S					
23		S	S					
24		S	S					
25		S	S					
26	S	S	S					
27	S	S	S					
28	S	S	S					
29	S	✕	S					
30	S	✕	S					
31	S	✕	S	✕				

CHART 14

Postmenstrual headaches, typically beginning on day 3 through 6 of the cycle, are not part of PMS. They do, however, occur in women who tend to be headache prone and who may also have some headaches premenstrually. Though these headaches are related to the menstrual cycle, little is known about why they occur when they do.

CHART 14

SYMPTOMS INITIALS

1. _Headache_ _H_

2. _____ _____

3. _____ _____

Menstruation: (M)

Date charting began: _____

MONTHS

	October	November	December					
1								
2								
3								
4		H						
5								
6								
7								
8								
9								
10								
11	(M)							
12	(M)	(M)						
13	(M) H	(M)	(M)					
14	(M) H	(M)	(M)					
15	H	(M) H	(M) H					
16	H	H	(M) H					
17	H	H	(M) H					
18		H	(M) H					
19			H					
20								
21								
22								
23								
24	H							
25	H							
26								
27								
28								
29								
30								
31		><						

CHART 15

This is the chart of a woman who has had a hysterectomy but whose
ovaries were not removed. Although there is no M for menses, the cyclic
symptoms are present. If this analysis is combined with a temperature
chart showing ovulation, the relationship between symptoms and ovulation becomes clearer.

CHART 15

SYMPTOMS   INITIALS

1. ___Symptoms_____   ___S___

2. _____   _____

3. _____   _____

Menstruation: ⊗

Date charting began: _____

MONTHS   *Hysterectomy*

	January	February	March	April	May			
1								
2			S					
3			S					
4			S		S			
5			S		S			
6			S		S			
7		S	S	S	S			
8	S	S	S	S	S			
9	S	S	S	S	S			
10	S	S		S	S			
11	S	S		S	S			
12	S	S		S	S			
13	S	S		S	S			
14	S			S	S			
15	S			S	S			
16	S			S	S			
17	S			S				
18	S			S				
19				S				
20								
21								
22								
23								
24								
25								
26								
27								
28								
29		✗		✗				
30		✗		✗				
31		✗		✗				

Patterns of Symptoms

The charts below show the most general patterns common to PMS in relation to the menstrual cycle. Typically when the cycle is longer, the symptoms begin later. It is usually assumed that a woman ovulates fourteen days prior to her next menstrual period, but sometimes women ovulate at other times.

CHART 16

In this case the symptoms appear at ovulation, then diminish or disappear, and then recur shortly before menses, ending with the onset of bleeding.

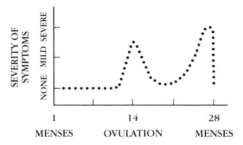

CHART 17

This chart illustrates gradually increasing premenstrual symptoms ending with menstruation.

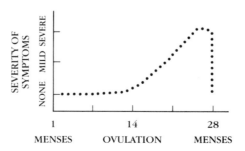

CHART 18

Here the symptoms become severe with ovulation and remain so until menses.

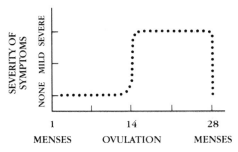

CHART 19

Some symptoms, especially headache, tend to extend into the menstrual time, through the first two or three days of the period.

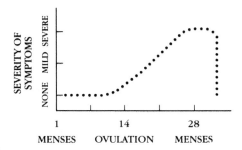

CHART 20

In cases of premenstrual magnification (PMM), symptoms are present throughout the cycle but are more severe premenstrually.

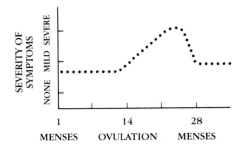

Ovulation

When it is not clear that symptoms are related to ovulation, as in long cycles, irregular cycles, or after hysterectomy when menses isn't present at all, you can chart ovulation. This is done by taking your temperature daily immediately upon awakening. A special thermometer, called a basal body thermometer, is useful for this because the temperature changes are measured in tenths of a degree, which are hard to read on a regular thermometer. Basal body thermometers can be purchased at any drugstore.

When basal body temperature is charted, ovulation is noted by a shift in temperature over several days. A woman's basal body temperature, or "resting" temperature, is slightly lower in the first part of her cycle and then rises one half to one degree after ovulation. Some women use temperature charting to determine when to avoid or have intercourse, since ovulation is the time of greatest fertility. In charting for PMS, all that is needed is a general sense of when ovulation has occurred, so don't worry if you miss a day or two.

Usually PMS is related to cycles in which ovulation has occurred, but it can also occur in the absence of ovulation, as when the ovaries have been removed. The following charts show the occurrence of ovulation:

CHART 21

Ovulation is noted by the drop and then sharp rise in temperature around day 14 or 15. Typically the temperature returns to its baseline approximately when menstruation begins.

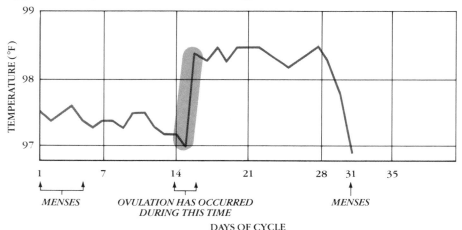

DAYS OF CYCLE

CHART 22

When the baseline average remains the same throughout the cycle, ovulation has not occurred. You can still get a period even if you have not ovulated. And you can have PMS in a cycle in which you have not ovulated.

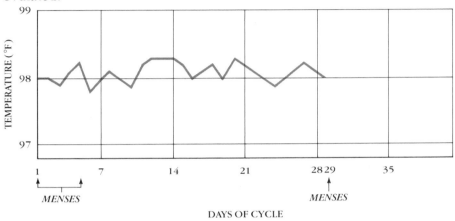

CHART 23

Ovulation usually occurs fourteen days **before** the next period, but sometimes women ovulate earlier or later than that. This chart represents a cycle in which ovulation occurred around day 9 or 10 of the cycle (the day of the cycle is counted from the first day of menstruation). If this woman has symptoms early in the month, around day 8 to 10, they may very well be premenstrual.

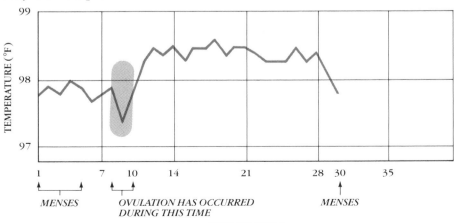

CHART 24

Here ovulation is occurring at the expected time, day 25, for a long cycle (forty days).

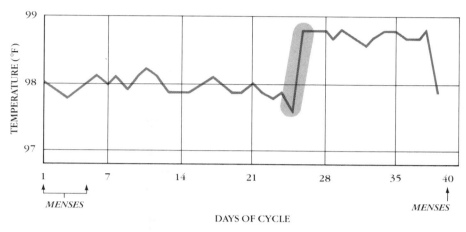

DAYS OF CYCLE

CHARTS 25 AND 26

Comparing temperature charts with symptom charts can be useful with irregular periods or when symptoms don't seem to make sense in terms of the cycle. The woman whose charts follow had symptoms beginning day 6 in January and day 16 in February. She then skipped a period in March, but had symptoms on Day 42 of the cycle, which began at the end of February. She then had her period 16 days after her symptoms began. In comparing the temperature charts she was keeping (Chart 26) with her symptom chart (Chart 25), it is clear that the onset of symptoms each month correlated with the days of the cycle on which she ovulated for each of those three cycles. The erratic presence of symptoms is explained by means of these charts. If, for example, ovulation had occurred around January 24–25, then the three days of symptoms earlier that month could not be attributed to PMS.

Remember also that the temperature chart is recording days of the cycle, while the symptoms are being charted by days of the month.

CHART 25

SYMPTOMS   INITIALS

1. _Symptoms_____ _S_

2. _____ _____   Menstruation: (M)

3. _____ _____   Date charting began: _____

MONTHS

	January	February	March	April					
1		(M)							
2		(M)							
3		(M)							
4		(M)							
5									
6									
7				S					
8				S					
9				S					
10				S					
11				S					
12				S					
13	(M)			S					
14	(M)			S					
15	(M)			S					
16	(M)	S		S					
17		S		S					
18	S	S		S					
19	S	S		S					
20	S	S		S					
21		S		S					
22		S		(M)					
23		S		(M)					
24		S		(M)					
25		(M)		(M)					
26		(M)							
27	S	(M)							
28	S	(M)							
29	S								
30	S								
31	S								

CHART 26

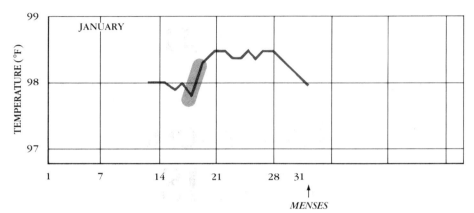

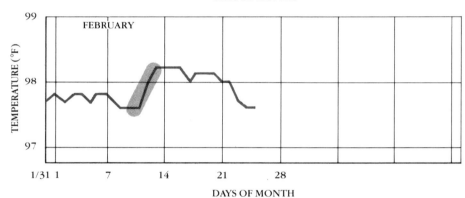

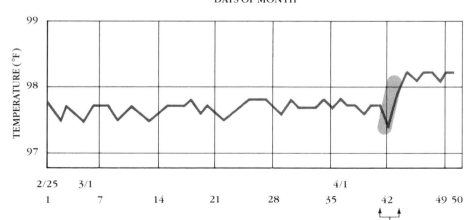

PART II

Treatment of PMS

CHAPTER 7

— ⊠ —

Treatment
of PMS

*I have not noticed any blues or crying feelings or spells.
It's apparently cleared up. It's not necessarily noticeable
because this is a normal way to feel day by day. It's only
if you feel bad that you notice that something's not right.*

*Recognition of PMS has had the most effect on me and
my life. I am now able to recognize feelings and relate them
to PMS and create a safer environment for myself. It's a
great improvement over paranoia.*

How do you treat PMS?

First, you treat a *woman* who has PMS. As overwhelming as PMS may
be at times, a woman is more than her dysfunctional condition. You treat
the PMS within the context of her whole life, including her life-style,
personal values, anxieties, support systems, and patience with the process.

Here are some general principles of PMS treatment:

• There is no one treatment for PMS which works for everyone. I do
  not know of any woman who has not obtained relief from some part
  of her PMS during the course of trying different programs, but the
  process can be a long one.

• PMS does not seem to like to go away. It often responds to treatment for a while and then returns, and this is true for all treatments. This is one of the reasons research is so difficult: without long-term studies we can only see the temporary results of any program.

- PMS treatment is often begun at a time of crisis for the woman and those around her. Therefore, it's important to sort out which symptoms are directly or indirectly related to the PMS, and which are unrelated but simultaneously present.

- Because of the emotional manifestations of PMS, its relief often creates changes in the woman's relationships to others. These shifts may not always be smooth. People adjust to their own illness, disability, and weakness, as do those around them. The readjustment to health and strength can be a challenge to everyone.

- Both the research concerning and the many treatments being suggested for PMS are fairly recent. More time is needed for them to be tested.

- Success with any PMS treatment can be erratic. The results may be inconsistent from time to time for the same person.

- PMS following tubal ligation or the use of oral contraceptives may be more difficult to treat than that following pregnancy or in cases of spontaneous onset.

- Medical practitioners may be less informed about PMS than a consumer who has read articles and a book or two on the subject. Unfortunately, there are medical practitioners who still do not know about or believe in the existence of PMS.

- Nothing is wrong with wanting total relief from all PMS symptoms, but it may not be possible.

- There are several stages in coming to terms with PMS as well as in treating it. They may occur in any order: denial of PMS, relief that PMS is "real," blame, anger, and/or acceptance.

- Compassion for one's self is necessary in dealing with PMS.

- PMS has been a secret because of silence; women's problems with it have been ignored. Women have thought themselves crazy and have been unable to support one another with their PMS problems because of that silence. The final solutions for PMS will come from the women who have hàd PMS and have shared their solutions.

- The historical lesson of PMS is that women have not been listened to and have allowed others to define their reality. It is important in treatment to keep careful records and notes as to what *feels* better or worse. If a treatment isn't working, it isn't because you imagine it isn't working.

Treatment of PMS falls into five major categories:

1. Life-style changes including diet, exercise, stress reduction, and relaxation exercises.

2. Nonprescription remedies such as vitamins, minerals, and food supplements.

3. Medications prescribed by medical practitioners—i.e., progesterone, antidepressants, diuretics, and others.

4. Alternative therapies such as acupuncture and massage.

5. Support systems and psychotherapy, including both leaderless support groups and individual or group psychotherapy.

The details of these treatments are in the following chapters.

CHAPTER 8

Diet and PMS

"Doctor, I'll do anything to get rid of these feelings."
"Then give up sugar and caffeine."
"Anything but that!"

Sometimes I think that women in our society are showing the effects of massive poisoning by substances that are part of our daily diet. In 1970 I didn't believe in hypoglycemia, the dangers of additives, or food allergies. I thought people who were concerned with those things were neurotic. I had been taught and had learned well the lessons of traditional medicine.

My ideas changed as I watched children and adults I know experience profound behavior changes in relation to the substances they took into their bodies. Traditional obstetrics had denied the role of diet and nutrition in pregnancy, but those who raised animals seemed to place great importance on diet for fetal development. I wondered why we didn't extend that awareness to humans. Was it our belief that our consciousness and spirit made us invulnerable to our bodies? As humans, we are both spirit and body, and balance between those parts is essential. Destruction of one can bring down the other.

We can also be addicted to substances that alter our moods and change our relationship to ourselves and our environment. We often eat foods to stimulate us, take drinks to slow us down, and swallow pills to do a variety of both.

The following dietary and food suggestions are based on my experience with hundreds of women whose PMS has been relieved as a result of major dietary changes. These guidelines are a result of my work with those women. I recommend that women with PMS try the diet described here. If it doesn't work in six months, then give it up. It may be healthy, but if it isn't helping your PMS and you aren't interested in a healthy diet for other reasons, then don't stay with it.

How to Change Your Diet

1. Determine your best approach to change. Think of going on a diet as though you were removing a Band-Aid. Some people remove them millimeter by millimeter, others with one quick rip. There is no right way to do it, but different approaches suit different people. There's going cold turkey or taking it slowly. Know your style and work with it. It's hard enough to change your diet without also trying to change the way you do things.

2. Acknowledge to yourself that changing your diet is difficult. Food represents more than sustenance. It represents security, style of life, reward, deprivation, ethnicity. Think of how it feels to be away from home and then to come home to the food you are used to cooking and eating. Food represents home, what is secure and familiar. None of this is easy to change.

3. Diet changes can be threatening to others around you. They may need to maintain that the way they eat is really okay. They may want to see you as someone who eats and drinks as they do. We think of people who offer free drugs to others to entice them into using them as deplorable. But have you ever tried telling someone you don't eat sugar anymore? Typical responses are similar to the way people used to respond to others who have stopped drinking alcohol. "Oh, one bite won't hurt," or "What's the matter with you!" or "You're neurotic," the latter either said out loud or implied—as I'm sure I did years ago. If you step back for a moment, you may wonder why anyone else should be so threatened

by what you eat. Why should others care, and if they do, is that your problem or theirs?

4. Try not to fight the change. Think about what you *can* eat and not what you *can't* eat. Make the change a challenge. Go to a library or store and get some cookbooks for ideas about how to prepare the foods on your diet so that they are appealing.

5. Give yourself four months of strict adherence to the diet. If you don't give it a real chance you will never know if it works. If after that time you see no results, then there is no reason why, in terms of PMS, you should stay with it. Often after several months of success on the diet you can "cheat" and try foods which you have cut out. Either they will make you sick and you won't try them again, or you will find that your body can now tolerate small amounts of foods that previously gave you difficulties.

6. The diet isn't effective if you try it only part of the month. It must be followed *all month long,* not just when you are premenstrual. It simply doesn't work to cut down only when you are premenstrual.

7. Expect to experience some withdrawal symptoms when you stop ingesting either sugar or caffeine, and expect a period of adjustment to whatever new substances you introduce into your diet. Withdrawal, especially from caffeine, produces lethargy and headaches that peak in about *ten days* and finally are relieved at about *two weeks.* Dietary change produces profound differences in how you feel and how you experience yourself.

8. The recommended diet for PMS is similar to but not exactly the same as typical diets for hypoglycemia. The PMS diet is more balanced, neither high protein nor low carbohydrate, and the balance of these can vary without creating difficulties.

9. The first dietary culprit in PMS appears to be sugar because it produces a drop in blood sugar. Alcohol, as a sugar, has the same effect.

Burning sugar (a simple carbohydrate) for fuel is like using newspaper for heat. It burns easily with a bright flame, then quickly dies, and you need more paper. Complex carbohydrates (as in whole grains and vegetables), protein, and fats are slow-burning, and like coal provide longer lasting and continual heat. Eat whole-grain foods rather than refined products.

Anything sweet can provoke a lowering of blood sugar, even noncaloric sweeteners. There is evidence that just looking at foods can provoke sugar absorption into cells, and so can just tasting something sweet. Like Pavlov's dogs who salivated for food at the sound of a bell, our bodies respond to look and taste, even in the absence of calories.

10. The second PMS offender is caffeine, probably because like sugar it stimulates insulin secretion, resulting in a rapid drop in blood sugar. Even decaffeinated beverages have some caffeine.

Some days I get several calls in a row from women whose PMS has disappeared when they gave up caffeine. One woman added, "I've always thought of myself as an anxious person, but you know, I think it was the caffeine all along."

11. If reading this much about diet has already produced panic, or if you are too depressed to make dietary changes, be kind to yourself; look to other remedies for PMS. Then as you begin to feel better you may be able to come back to the diet, or if other remedies do not work, you may be forced to come back and to pay attention to your diet. If that happens, your motivation will be stronger.

12. The diet for PMS is not a weight reduction diet. Neither losing nor gaining weight will help PMS. It is possible to lose *or* gain weight on the diet for PMS depending on the choices and quantities of foods eaten.

13. There is much controversy about salt limitation with respect to PMS. Except in cases in which women are aware of bloating after salt consumption, there does not seem to be any reason to limit salt in PMS. What bloating does occur is primarily a redistribution of water that takes place whether or not there is increased salt intake. In fact, there can be as much water retention following carbohydrate consumption as following salt consumption. The water accumulation blamed on the potato chips may be from the M&M's as well.

14. Eat frequently—that is, small quantities every two to three hours—rather than consuming large meals with fasting between. The snacks need not be elaborate or large, just enough to keep the internal furnace burning steadily and evenly.

15. A late-night high-protein snack that provides some fuel for all-night burning can minimize or prevent early morning symptoms.

16. As you read through the recommended diet you will find that it may contradict other diets, including some designed for PMS. However, the following food guidelines have successfully worked for many women with PMS. Women with specific allergies to some food will naturally have to modify these lists.

Before You Panic . . . What Can You Eat?

MEATS, POULTRY, FISH: Large quantities of animal protein and fat are not particularly healthy. Diets high in animal protein have been linked to cancer of the breast, colon, and uterus, as well as to heart disease. However, they need not be omitted if PMS is what you are treating. Be aware, though, that some women develop sweet cravings after eating a meal heavy in animal protein.

Especially as you begin the transition to a new diet, it is important to hold on to as many familiar foods as possible and then make further changes if you want to in the future. It's taken twenty or thirty or forty years of habit to create the diet you now have. Don't expect to be able to change it all at once. Concentrate initially on those substances that need to be omitted in order to bring PMS symptoms under control. Then you may want to improve the general quality of your diet over time.

You may eat the following:

beef	*pork*
chicken	*shellfish*
fish	*turkey*
lamb	

These may be prepared fried (unless you are watching calories), or baked, broiled, poached, steamed, or stewed.

VEGETABLES: These may be eaten in any quantity at any time. If you are concerned about your weight, avoid large quantities of those with higher caloric content.

artichokes

asparagus

avocado

bean sprouts

beans, green

beet greens

beets

broccoli

brussels sprouts

cabbage

carrots

cauliflower

celery

chicory

chick-peas (garbanzos)

chinese cabbage

collards

corn

cucumber

eggplant

endive

escarole

kale

leeks

lentils

lettuce

lima beans

mushrooms

navy beans

okra

onion

parsley

parsnip

peas

peppers, red and green

potato

pumpkin

radishes

rhubarb

rutabaga

spinach

scallions

snow peas

squash

string beans

sweet potato

tomatoes

turnip

watercress

yams

zucchini

GRAINS, BEANS, PEAS: Eat plenty of whole grains or products made from whole grains. For instance, wheat can be eaten as flour or as steamed or boiled wheat berries. Likewise, rice can be in flour form or as whole rice. Corn can be used as meal or as whole kernels. Do not forget popcorn, an easily prepared snack food.

barley

buckwheat

bulgur

corn

lentils

millet

oats (and oatmeal)

peanuts

rice

rye

soybeans and soybean products,
    including tofu and tempeh

triticale

wheat

NUTS AND SEEDS: These are nutritious but tend to be high in calories.

almonds	*pignolia*
Brazil nuts	*pistachio*
cashews	*pumpkin seeds*
coconut	*sunflower seeds*
filberts	*walnuts*
pecans	

FRUITS: The only problem with fruits is that in large quantities they may act as a sugar substitute and produce the same effects. Enjoy your fruit but limit it to about three servings a day. (A serving is generally 1/2 cup fruit or 4 ounces of juice.) Fruit is better eaten with a meal; alone, as a snack, it is more inclined to act like candy. You may have the following fruits or unsweetened juices made from them:

apples	*lemon*
applesauce (unsweetened)	*mangoes**
apricots	*melons*
bananas	*nectarines*
blackberries	*orange*
blueberries	*papaya**
cantaloupe	*peach*
cherries*	*pears*
cider	*persimmon*
cranberries	*pineapple**
dates*	*plums*
figs*	*prunes**
grapefruit	*raisins**
grapes	*tangerines*
honeydew	*watermelon*

DAIRY PRODUCTS: Other than considerations of cutting down on animal fats, there is no PMS-related reason to avoid dairy products. You may eat the following:

butter	*cottage cheese*
cheese, hard or soft	*eggs*
cream cheese	*farmer cheese*

Fruits marked with * are especially sweet and should be limited to one serving a day. A cup and a half of cherries defeats the purpose of avoiding sweets.

milk, whole or skim   *sour cream*
ricotta cheese   *yogurt*

WATER: This is one of the most important substances you take into your body. It constitutes the major part of your cellular makeup. Drink water freely. Far from causing bloating, water actually acts as a diuretic. In order for the kidneys to excrete water, they must add salt to it, so drinking plain water leads to excretion of the water plus salt. The bloating of PMS is related to redistribution of water and to the body's holding of water. It is not related to water consumption.

What You Cannot Eat

SUGAR, HONEY, MOLASSES, ARTIFICIAL SWEETENER, MALT, CORN SYRUP, ETC.: In other words, if it tastes sweet, you cannot have it. The reason for omitting even artificial sweeteners is that, as mentioned before, the body reacts to them as if they were sugar. Only after they are absorbed does it matter whether they carry calories or not. The body's basic reactions to them are based on taste. The only exception to this rule is that most breads need some sweetening agent to make the yeast rise. That small amount of sugar, in a nonsweet bread or roll, is permissible.

CAFFEINE: This category includes decaffeinated coffees and teas, for even decaf drinks have some caffeine in them. Caffeine reacts by its presence alone and not solely by amount. Adding caffeine is like adding red dye to clear water; even one drop makes the water red. Many drops make it redder, but even a touch produces the color. Even decaf has enough caffeine to produce a blood sugar reaction. The following beverages and drugs contain caffeine: coffee, tea, colas, diet colas, chocolate, many painkillers and cold preparations, some of which also contain alcohol. Herbal teas and grain beverages are excellent substitutes. So is bottled spring water with a twist of lemon or lime.

WHITE-FLOUR PRODUCTS: Pasta, white bread, and other foods made with highly refined substances should be omitted. It is very difficult to get whole-wheat bread made without any white flour, which is why I specify no white flour *products* rather than no white flour. The pasta you eat should be made with other grains and starches, such as whole wheat, soy, and jerusalem artichoke flours.

ALCOHOL: This should be totally avoided as it contains sugar and is a central nervous system depressant.

NICOTINE: This should be avoided, but it is the least important of the PMS related dietary restrictions. This is not a defense of smoking, and in fact smoking remains dangerous to your health in general, but it is possible to rid oneself of PMS and still smoke . . . and then, one hopes, be able to conquer that addiction later on.

Specific Foods to Be Avoided

JUNK FOOD, ICE CREAM, CAKE, CANDY, PREPARED FOODS WHICH HAVE SUGAR AS A MAJOR INGREDIENT, WHITE BREAD, DOUGH-NUTS, SODAS (INCLUDING DIET SODAS), ALCOHOL, NICOTINE, COFFEE AND CAFFEINE-CONTAINING FOODS, "DECAFFEINATED" COFFEE, CHOCOLATE

About Addictions

Admittedly, getting rid of addictions is difficult. The first step is to recognize that you are addicted. The best way to know if you are addicted is to notice your reaction to being told you should give something up. If you get a sick feeling in your gut, or anxiety, or if you tell yourself you could give it up if you had to but you're not sure you have to, then you are probably hooked.

The second way to know if you are hooked is by trying to stop. If you feel worse—depressed or irritable, for example—and believe that some substance will make you feel better, then you are hooked on that substance. And you probably will feel better, at least until the next time your level of that substance runs low.

If you spend your time fantasizing about a certain food or substance, you are hooked on it. If you dream of candy bars and coffee, your body is probably telling you it is missing them. It is amazing that our society condemns drug addicts when most Americans are unable to abstain from coffee or sugar for even a week.

One cup of coffee in the morning still constitutes an addiction and still affects your PMS. Try making it weaker and weaker, or have half a cup of coffee and half a cup of herbal tea or grain beverage at first. You will be amazed at how you become accustomed to the new drinks as they gain the importance of your former morning coffee.

Others may not be supportive of your attempt to give up these foods. They may react with open hostility and cold resistance or by placing sweets in view around the house. Children are especially threatened by changes in food, but so are adults. Eating meals together, breaking bread, is a basic part of what we do together as humans, and changes in those patterns can create deep insecurities. It has been said that children equate sugar with love. They may not be the only ones.

There is no one cookbook specific for this PMS diet, but using many of the current health food cookbooks and leaving out such things as sugar or sweetener in traditional recipes can result in tasty and nutritious eating. (Some books are listed in the bibliography.)

When you first try to follow this diet it may seem that there is nothing to eat; go back to the foods listed in the section on what you can eat. There is a lot there.

Cutting sugar and caffeine out of your diet does not require prior consultation with your physician. We have become quite accustomed to the warning that we should see a doctor before making dietary changes, but what is presented here is a basic healthy diet with a few toxic substances missing. It may be, instead, that we should consult someone *before* consuming sugar, caffeine, alcohol, and other refined products, but it's certainly not necessary as a prerequisite to giving them up.

> *It's wonderful to finally have relief from my depression and moodiness. It's the result of the diet. All symptoms are practically gone except withdrawal, and I can talk myself through because I know I'm premenstrual.*

CHAPTER 9

Exercise

EXERCISE CAN HELP PROVIDE a sense of well-being as well as an outlet for excess energy, and it is an effective way of relieving body tension. Many women are too fatigued or depressed to exercise when they are premenstrual. Also, because of bloating, they are especially prone to feeling bad about their bodies. It is therefore important to establish an exercise regimen that can be sustained *throughout the menstrual cycle.*

Exercise can become a habit and can even become addictive. Many women find that once they get a routine of exercise established, they feel lost, unsettled, or irritable on days when they cannot continue it. One woman began walking every morning before breakfast. It became her time to be alone, to think, and to move her body. As she realized the importance of her walking, she became better able to protect her time. Looking back, she described how she had felt:

> *I felt so bad about myself I didn't think I deserved the time to exercise.*

Exercise has two components. One is the physical activity, and the other is the taking of time to care for one's body and one's self. Both are necessary if exercise is to help PMS. Being on your feet all day does not constitute exercise, nor does doing housework or even construction work. Those activities do require movement of the body, but without the environment that allows this movement to be translated into a self-nurturing or self-development experience. Doing housework does not decrease depression or lead to an increase in self-esteem, but taking time for a walk, even if the total energy expenditure is less, will combat depression and enhance self-confidence and esteem. A peace of mind must be present for the exercise to produce its beneficial effects. Aerobic exercise can be fine but not if there is also a two-year-old tugging at your skirt or falling on your stomach.

Exercise must be

> *pleasurable*   *thirty minutes at least*
> *daily*   *uninterrupted*

It matters less what the particular exercise is and more that it provides some *pleasure.* If it does not, you will find it almost impossible to be motivated sufficiently to do the exercise when you are premenstrual.

The exercise must also be daily. The body can come to count on this regular release of tension, and as a result anxieties may begin to be stored until that time each day.

For women trying to control weight, exercising in the morning leads to more weight loss than exercise done later in the day. Morning exercise seems to set the body's metabolic rate higher so that more calories are burned off during the day.

What matters for relief of PMS is not the number of miles walked or jogged, but the *quality* of that experience. The pleasure and benefit of reading books cannot be measured by the number of words read. It is an experience that can only be measured by the enhancement of your sense of well-being.

It is important to differentiate exercise for cardiovascular fitness or weight loss from exercise for PMS. Walking to work or using stairs instead of elevators will enhance both fitness and weight loss but may do nothing for PMS. It is really the combination of movement and *the sense of well-being* that is helpful for PMS.

Exercises

WALKING: Strolling or racewalking both qualify, as well as speeds intermediate between the two. Walking to work helps for fitness or weight loss, but rarely includes the necessary ingredient of peacefulness. For exercise to be helpful for PMS it must include the commitment to take time out for oneself. Taking a walk before the day begins, at lunchtime, after work, or after others come home to relieve women at home with children are all ways of releasing tension and moving one's body beneficially. Walking also promotes bone strength, and it can be done outdoors, in cities, and in rural areas.

JOGGING: Jogging is a popular form of exercise but is dependent on weather conditions, except for those people close to an indoor track. Speed isn't important; what does matter is achieving that sense of well-being and then *maintaining* it.

SWIMMING: Swimming is excellent exercise that can be done either outdoor or indoors depending on the time of year and your proximity to pools. For many women it provides a time when they cannot be interrupted and thus combines body movement with time to oneself. Again, the number of laps are not at issue here, but rather the quality of the experience. It would be so much easier if one could prescribe a certain number of laps or miles that would relieve PMS. The experience is what counts, though, not the distance or the exertion.

BIKING AND USING EXERCISE BIKES: the combination of the two, which allows for daily exercise independent of weather, can be exhilarating. Riding an exercise bike can also be boring, but it can be combined with reading, listening to music, or other activities.

AEROBIC EXERCISING AND DANCING: This can be done in classes, in front of the TV, with tapes, or with some combination of the above. Few women can or want to go to classes daily, but a combination of classes and home tapes can become a daily routine.

Exercises such as dancing, horseback riding, ice skating, skiing, squash, tennis, volleyball, and others can also be pleasurable and useful. They can be part of your routine, but since they are rarely *daily* exercises they should be mixed with others so that you are sure to do something each day.

Planning Exercise

1. Start your exercise program when you are *not* premenstrual. Take advantage of the good feeling that begins with or shortly after your period commences. In the midst of PMS not much feels good, so don't expect to implement life-style changes then.

2. Give yourself a month or two to establish your regular exercise program. Begin by listing those exercises you might like, those you've always enjoyed, those you didn't enjoy before but might like to try again, those you've always wanted to try but for which you haven't had the time, energy, or motivation.

3. Try different exercises during the first months. For instance, take a long walk one day, swim at a local Y another. If you begin by thinking, "This is what I'm going to have to do each day," you may be defeating yourself at the start. Try jogging one day, not for distance, but just to see how it feels. Check TV listings for exercise shows you can watch and participate in at home. Take advantage of health clubs that let you use their facilities once or twice before you have to join.

4. Begin to look at yourself as someone who exercises and is simply looking for the right form to use. Imagine yourself dancing, running, or sitting on an exercycle.

5. Begin an exercise journal. The following pages may be helpful to you in organizing your approach to your exercise. Try them, but if keeping such records is stressful, then proceed without them. (See the appendix for additional copies of these forms.)

Exercise Journal

EXERCISE I LIKE	EXERCISE TO RETRY	EXERCISE I ALWAYS WANTED TO TRY

FIVE EXERCISES TO TRY THIS MONTH

1. Exercise _____ How I will do it _____
_____

2. Exercise _____ How I will do it _____
_____

3. Exercise _____ How I will do it _____
_____

4. Exercise _____ How I will do it _____
_____

5. Exercise _____ How I will do it _____
_____

FILL-IN EXERCISES While I am trying new forms of exercise I will use the following exercises on a daily basis so that each day I do something.

_____
_____
_____
_____

Weekly Exercise Journal

Use this form to keep track of the exercises you are doing. It will be interesting to see how, over time, your ability and pleasure increase.

Week of _____

	S	M	T	W	T	F	S
EXERCISE							
TIME OF DAY							
HOW LONG							
HOW IT FELT							
WHAT NEEDS TO BE CHANGED							

CHAPTER 10

Stress and PMS

"The Body Takes on the Pain of the Soul"

Stress does not cause PMS, but it can add to premenstrual symptoms and to premenstrual magnification of symptoms. PMS, however, can be a cause of stress.

What is stress? It is a state of tension with both emotional and physiological manifestations. The body's response to stress is to stimulate the hypothalamus (the "conductor" of PMS) and to alter brain-wave activity. Feeling stressed or having a physical reaction to stress is not an act of conscious will. It is a physiological and chemical alteration of the brain affecting the hypothalamus, which integrates and mediates neurological and endocrine responses. Since this area already appears to be dysfunctional in PMS, the addition of stress stimuli can make the symptoms worse. On an emotional level, the combination of PMS, in which there is often an inner pull toward quiet or even withdrawal, and *constant stress* add to the confusion, tension, and occasional panic of the syndrome.

So what do you do? The first thing is to identify areas of major stress. People are often afraid to acknowledge stressful situations because they fear that they are then supposed to give them up, but this is not necessarily so. Some stresses are useful. When not incapacitating, stress can lead to increased performance and creativity. Without deadlines, for example, we would all probably accomplish little. And stress can be an important component in challenge. The object is not necessarily to give up stress but to have some control over it and to be able to choose which stresses one wants to handle and which one would rather let go of. Some stresses we may not be able to do anything about at this time in our lives, but even coming to terms with that reality can be helpful.

Looking at Stress

Stress can arise from any of the following sources. It can be useful to look at each and ask yourself these questions:

1. Work:
    What is the work I am doing?
    Do I enjoy it?
    Would I rather be doing something else?
    How important is that something else to me?

2. Health:
    Do I have health problems other than my PMS?
    Am I satisfied with my body?
    Am I at war with my body?
    What would I like to change?
    What do I think I might be able to change?

3. Economics:
    Am I satisfied with my present economic life?
    Is it different from the circumstances of my childhood?
    Is there disparity of economic goals within my home?
    Do I have control over my financial situation?
    *Am I comfortable with the way in which money is
        handled in my life?*

4. Primary adult relationships:
    *What is/are my primary relationships like, with my husband, lover,
        partner, parent?*
    What are the difficult areas?
    What is most gratifying?

For the moment do I think I am basically satisfied in each relationship?

5. Children: Children themselves can cause stress, and so can the work involved in caring for them. Added to that is the stress women feel in protecting the children from their own premenstrual mood swings and anger.

    What are the good and the difficult times with my children?
    Do I feel alone? Supported?
    Do I think they are difficult children?
    Do I think I am difficult as a parent?
    What do I need to make my life with them better?
    Am I in conflict with others about the children—i.e. with spouse, parents, friends?

6. Friendships:
    Do I have a network of supportive friends?
    Has that network changed recently? Have I isolated myself?
    Have I crowded my life with friends to avoid being alone?

7. Self:
    Am I comfortable with myself, when I'm not in the midst of PMS?
    What pleases me about myself?
    What might I wish to change?

8. Time:
    How do I relate to the concept of time?
    Does the word "time" make me panic because there never seems to be enough?
    Which of my time stresses seem temporary?
    Which seem a permanent part of my life?
    How would I like to change my relationship to time?

9. Being alone:
    Do I have time alone?
    Am I afraid to be alone?
    Is there support for me to have time alone?
    Do I believe I deserve it?

10. Spirituality:
    What are my present beliefs?

Have they changed?
Am I satisfied with changes in my sense of spirituality?
Is there conflict in my family regarding spirituality?
Do I give room to this part of my life?
How is my spirituality affected by PMS?

> *I consider myself a very religious person. One of the worst parts about having PMS has been that I sometimes lose my faith when I am in the worst PMS. I can't find anything to believe in. I'm just miserable and I want to get angry with God. I try to look at what I am supposed to learn and why I am suffering, but I can't find any meaning in it, except that I understand other people's pain more.*

PMS at times occurs in a woman's life when she is undergoing deep questioning of her identity, purpose, and belief systems. The crisis of body dysfunction accompanies the crisis of being. I have watched them develop together and have seen them resolve themselves simultaneously.

Methods of Stress Reduction

Stress reduction requires first that you recognize stress exists and then that you desire to lessen it. There is a high that comes with stressful living, as well as a high associated with living from crisis to crisis. Trying to reduce stress without recognizing this can lead to failure. The intent to lessen stress is helpful in itself, but looking for the perfect way to do it or expecting to become stress-free in a week can create even more stress.

Reducing stress is more than learning to forget it or to stop getting so upset. Few of us are free of the voices in our heads that constantly give us instructions. What we are dealing with here is a more profound alteration in your way of being, a shift in how you experience yourself and your environment. Achieving that goal is not easy.

Relaxation and stress reduction do not happen by trying harder to make them happen. What is required is the opposite of learning a language, where the more you practice, the more you learn. Here, the harder you try to relax, the less you are apt to succeed.

It is important to look at stress reduction as a "one day at a time" process. There is always stress, there are always stressful events, but recognizing what is outside oneself versus what is within your own control makes PMS, as well as much of life, easier. Stress reduction is not something one simply does daily for a particular amount of time. It is a way of approaching one's life. It's like a shift in background color of a painting, or a change in a camera lens. It is the creation of a new way of being.

Stress-reduction techniques (a long phrase for what is supposed to make life easier) are most useful if they become integrated into your life on a regular basis. Unlike exercises that demand a separate time, these methods can often be done in ten-minute intervals at work, at the end of a long line at the bank, or even in the midst of a traffic jam when remembering to focus or release or just to relax your muscles can have a tremendously beneficial effect on your sense of peace.

Try to schedule a regular time each day (however brief it may be) in which to practice some of these methods. Post reminders to yourself to use the techniques in strategic places (on your mirror or on the refrigerator door, for example). Most important, though, is to recognize that inner change does not occur overnight, and it rarely happens in an even, steady progression.

Begin to try out various ways of reducing stress. There are many magazine articles about stress reduction, many books and cassette programs, and many classes being offered at schools, Y's, and other places.

Look at the following suggestions for ways of stress reduction, live with them, think about them, try them, but most of all, let yourself begin to see yourself as a person who will be living with *less stress.* That's not to say that life will go easily, but the aim is to experience stresses without being eaten up inside or lashing out at others.

A WORD ABOUT THESE METHODS: They seem simple—*Breathe . . . Find a quiet place . . . Meditate . . . Let go . . . Imagine a peaceful scene*—but they are not. As with diet, one doesn't change a lifetime of patterning in a day or after a few paragraphs. Presented below is information *about* some of these methods, but not instructions on how to practice them. To try to teach these methods here (particularly the meditation, releasing, focusing, relaxation techniques, and self-hypnosis) would be doing a disservice to you and to these methods. I recommend instead that you look at some of the books and tapes. (Some are listed in the bibliography.)

As you begin to learn these methods, you need to make room for them in your life, and to make room for the changes they will create. Learn several ways of using these techniques, including when you might not want to use them, and what to do when they don't seem to be working. Some people become anxious when they begin to try these new things. Don't give up, but also don't force yourself. In some instances you may want to seek out someone who can personally guide you in this work.

MEDITATION: Many forms of meditation can help induce a sense of inner peace and an increased ability to deal with stressful situations. Meditation is a simple mental technique which allows the mind to calm down. It has at times been associated with religious and cultic activities, but there are now newer methods of meditating that can easily be learned by anyone, and that require no affinity to a group or belief system. Meditation simply consists of creating quiet time in which to sit or walk alone, and then silently repeating a soothing sound or word in a special manner. Some people can meditate while swimming or jogging.

RELEASING, FOCUSING: These two recent methods of dealing with one's own hair-trigger reaction to stress can be useful for PMS. They consist of simple techniques for teaching oneself to let go of overinvolvement in the outcome of a particular problem so you can cope more calmly and effectively. Again, the object is not to float into a state of nirvana at the sign of stressful events or to drop out, but rather to learn ways in which you can peacefully and with satisfaction survive some of the unavoidable stress and chaos of our lives.

SELF-HYPNOSIS: This is a process of self-suggestion one can learn either from a practitioner or from reading books on the subject. It is especially useful for breaking habits and dealing with cravings.

RELAXATION TECHNIQUES: These are methods of directly relaxing the body. They can be done by concentrating on breathing, by attending to body muscles and their tension or relaxation, or by imagining peaceful scenes, a process often called visualizing. There are many varieties of these techniques. Read about them and try what seems appealing.

YOGA: Yoga involves both breathing and stretching exercises that many people find relaxing and stress-reducing. There are several books that can be useful for someone trying yoga alone, and in many communities there are responsible yoga classes which one can attend. There are also yoga classes on TV, usually early in the morning or late at night. Yoga exercises can put undue strain on the body. It's important to proceed slowly and to get expert advice.

MASSAGE: Regular massage, especially during the premenstrual period, may provide physical relaxation, which in turn reduces emotional tension and thus lessens stress reactions. I sometimes think of PMS as a brick wall that must be broken through each month for the woman to feel relief. Some force is necessary to overcome the emotional state, and that force can be medication, a bout of tears, an angry outburst, or sometimes a good massage.

EXPRESSIVE ARTS: Drawing, music, writing, knitting, needlework, baking bread—all can give you the sense of peace that goes beyond the moment and affects general mood and coping ability.

JOURNAL WRITING: Keeping a journal requires some privacy and some time to oneself. There are many ways of using this useful technique. It can simply represent a way of silently screaming at what bothers you, or it can include a process of thinking out loud but alone. It also provides an ongoing record for looking back as you begin to take hold of your PMS and your life in general; and it can be an expression of your fantasy and of longings. All these uses are healthy and can lead to the reduction of stress.

Here are some ways to start a journal. As with exercise, the form often matters less than what it comes to mean to you as an experience.

- Use a blank book, preferably one that you find appealing.
- Try using a dated journal. The dates on each page can be an impetus to write, but they can also be oppressive, so watch your own reaction and modify your journal writing accordingly.
- Be flexible about what you want to cover each day. For instance, your journal can describe your emotions, your exercise, the food you are eating, stresses, feelings about relationships, work, time, aspirations, resentments, support (present or absent), what you are doing for yourself today, what you are learning about yourself at this time.
- Go back to your journal when you are not premenstrual and reassess your feelings, reactions, what you were doing for/against yourself. The "Bad Day Report" at the end of this chapter can be useful. Date it and note the day of your last period. You will want to know if this bad day was premenstrual or not. Describe the day, and then a week or so later go back and see if it now looks different. What can you learn now about the stress, your reaction to it, or your PMS?

Under stress it is easy to forget everything you know about coping mechanisms. Stress reactions can interfere with good judgment, and at those moments when life seems out of control, you may not remember your stress reduction techniques. In spite of all your reading and efforts, you may have setbacks at times of crisis. The next time of crisis, though, may be a bit easier because of what you have learned. And the next easier still.

Bad Day Report

DATE _____   LAST PERIOD _____

DAY OF CYCLE _____

What happened?

Foods eaten (note also any long stretches without eating):

Exercise:

Current stresses:

Review of the day several days later: How does the day look in retro-
spect? Are issues raised that still may be important? Was the diet that day
a healthy one? What have you learned?

CHAPTER 11

Vitamins, Minerals, and Oil of Evening Primrose

VITAMINS ARE HELPFUL IN CERTAIN SITUATIONS, and specific vitamins have been useful in PMS. They should not, however, be taken casually. People often assume that vitamins are safe because they are sold without prescription. In fact very little research has been done regarding their safety. People who would seriously question the medications prescribed by a physician will often take lots of vitamins with little or no hesitation.

Vitamin B_6

Vitamin B_6 at doses of 200 to 500 milligrams daily has relieved symptoms of depression and bloating for some women, and I have found this to be true in my practice. In 1983, however, one report indicated severe neurological side effects when women ingested B_6 at dosages of 2,000 milligrams per day or more, without taking any other B vitamins. B_6 should be taken along with the entire B complex, never alone. Because both practitioners and patients remain unsure of the safe dosage, it is recommended that the maximum dosage be 500 milligrams per day and that it be balanced by adding the other B vitamins, such as are obtainable in a standard B complex tablet.

Undesirable side effects of B$_6$ include headache, dizziness, nausea, and restless sleep or nightmares. If these symptoms appear, the B$_6$ should be decreased, and if they persist, the vitamin should be discontinued altogether. B$_6$ should be taken with food to avoid gastric upset.

Calcium/Magnesium

The correct use of calcium and magnesium for PMS is quite confusing. Calcium and magnesium, in a ratio of 2 to 1, have traditionally been used to treat premenstrual and menstrual cramping. The dosage suggested is usually about 500 milligrams calcium to 250 milligrams magnesium. However, there is some evidence that women with PMS have a deficiency of magnesium and therefore need more magnesium than this amount. To further complicate the issue, calcium is believed to *deplete* the body's magnesium. Researchers involved in magnesium study often advocate that the calcium/magnesium ratio be reversed—that is, be 1 to 2. One way to deal with this confusion can be to vary the dosage with the symptoms. Women who have premenstrual and menstrual cramping but without other PMS symptoms can take calcium/magnesium at 2 to 1, and those who have PMS without cramping can take it in a 1 to 2 ratio. Those with PMS cramping and other premenstrual symptoms take equal amounts of calcium and magnesium.

"PMS Vitamins"

There are now a number of vitamin combinations being sold in health food stores, clinics, and pharmacies for PMS. Most are high in B$_6$ as well as magnesium. Whether any one of these is superior to another is unclear, since much of the vitamin research has been conducted by the people who also market the products.

Potassium

Potassium, like sodium, or common table salt, is a salt necessary for the body's cells to function properly. Often, however, sodium and potassium are inversely related in body functioning. For instance, as the body retains sodium, it excretes, or puts out in the urine, the potassium. As one salt moves into the cells, the other moves out. Low potassium can be a cause of fatigue, and for that reason, foods rich in potassium should be eaten during the premenstrual time. Too high concentrations of potassium can be dangerous, and can cause heart irregularities and even death. For that reason, one should not take potassium pills or supplements except under medical supervision.

Potassium can be safely and easily obtained by eating many unprocessed foods such as grains, nuts and fresh vegetables. (Isn't it amazing how the same foods keep cropping up whenever health is being considered!)

Foods high in potassium are

- Nuts: almonds, Brazil nuts, chestnuts, coconut, filberts, peanuts, pecans, sesame seeds, sunflower seeds, and walnuts.
- Vegetables: artichokes, avocados, beans, beet greens, broccoli, brussels sprouts, carrots, celery, swill chard, collards, kale, mustard greens, parsley, parsnips, potatoes, spinach, squash, yams.
- Grains: wheat, buckwheat, rice.
- Fruits: apples, bananas, cantaloupes, dates, figs, grapefruit, lemons, oranges, raisins.
- Kelp and garlic.

As with the other dietary guidelines given for PMS, these are basically healthy foods, so eating them does not require medical consultation or supervision.

Oil of Evening Primrose

The evening primrose plant is a North American wildflower whose seeds contain an oil that has been found helpful in PMS. The oil contains an essential fatty acid, gamma-linolenic acid, which, incidentally, is also found in human breast milk. Several studies have shown oil of evening primrose to be effective for symptoms of PMS, especially for breast tenderness and swelling. In some cases it has also benefited the emotional symptoms.

Since this preparation is still being studied for PMS, the exact dosage has not yet been established. It is usually prepared in capsules of 0.5 gram to be taken three to four times daily throughout the month. If the first month's treatment is not successful, then during the second month the dosage is increased to six capsules per day. If still necessary, the third month the dosage may be raised to eight capsules a day. After that, it should be possible to cut down on the number taken so that you can eventually take only one a day and this only during the premenstrual time of the cycle.

Oil of evening primrose should be ingested with food, since by itself it may cause gastric irritation. Allergic reactions to this oil are rare but occasionally occur. Although oil of evening primrose is used for skin problems, it may itself cause skin irritations. The only known contraindication is in women with alcohol-induced migraine headaches.

The preparation is available without prescription and is widely sold in pharmacies and health food stores. Reading the label is important, however, as some products now being sold actually contain *other* noneffective oils rather than genuine oil of evening primrose.

CHAPTER 12

✖

Progesterone

For ten years I was living a hell on earth, ashamed of myself because of the way I was acting. But I couldn't help it. I would hide in my room, yell, and hit out at my husband. I tried to kill myself twice. Now that I have been taking progesterone I have not had any problems for two years. I feel normal again.

Progesterone is not a self-help treatment. I discuss it here because, as yet, so little is known about it in the medical community that a woman considering its use must first learn how to use it, what difficulties to expect or be aware of, and what potential risks exist.

Progesterone therapy for PMS has been used in England by Dr. Katharina Dalton since 1948 and in the United States since 1981. By now, thousands of women have taken progesterone for PMS and have reported good results with it even after other treatments have failed. However, there has been little controlled research as to either its usefulness or its long-term safety.

The progesterone used for the treatment of PMS must be distinguished from the progesterone-like substances (progestogens) that are used in birth control pills and to control irregular bleeding. The former (derived from soybeans and yams) is of the same chemical formulation as the progesterone secreted by your ovaries; the latter has some proges-

terone-like actions, but also has other effects that unfortunately can make
PMS worse. In fact, one of the reasons for the lack of physician enthusiasm for progesterone in the United States is a confusion between these
two substances. When progesterone treatment was first introduced here,
many doctors gave women progestogens instead of progesterone. They
believed that what they were giving was more convenient, since it was
a pill, and "just as good." When their treatment was unsuccessful, they
then assumed that *progesterone* doesn't work.

Unfortunately this confusion between the two compounds still exists.
One way to tell the two apart is that progesterone *cannot* be given in pill
form; progestogens are not given either rectally or vaginally.

> *I was sick on birth control pills. I was depressed almost
> the entire three years I took them. I put on fifteen pounds
> and it seemed I had a headache all the time. When I heard
> about progesterone I assumed it wouldn't work, but in my
> case it turned out to be just the opposite.*

Progesterone, when it works, seems to prevent or alleviate premenstrual symptoms so that the woman feels normal or "like herself." It does
not usually produce the drowsiness or fogginess characteristic of tranquilizers. The woman who benefits from progesterone is not particularly
aware of being on a medication. When the hormone loses its effectiveness, after several hours or a day, she may suddenly become aware again
of her PMS.

Although progesterone can be very effective in reducing extremes of
emotions premenstrually, it has no effect on the same emotional states
if the woman is not premenstrual. A woman on progesterone therapy
had a fight with her boyfriend a few days after her period. He turned
to her and said, "Why don't you take some of your medicine?" She
replied sharply, "This isn't PMS. I'm angry about our relationship, and
progesterone won't cure that." Since she was not premenstrual, the
progesterone did not affect her anger.

> *I can tell when it's me and when it's my PMS. Being
> angry when I know I'm right makes me feel good, but being
> angry when I know it's just me makes me feel sick inside.*

Progesterone tends to work against the latter but not the former.

Progesterone Therapy

1. Progesterone therapy sometimes takes months to work because of the need to adjust timing and dose to suit the symptoms, which may vary from cycle to cycle.

2. When progesterone works well, it provides immediate relief, within an hour. On the other hand, it sometimes gives only slight relief, in which case you have to decide whether to try using larger doses. Even when it relieves PMS totally, progesterone may not work as well the second month it is used. Often after the first seemingly miraculous success, it takes several more months to achieve the same results.

3. Progesterone is most commonly used vaginally as a suppository or rectally as a suppository or a suspension. It can also be used sublingually (under the tongue) or by deep intramuscular injection. Some women absorb progesterone better rectally and some vaginally; sublingual progesterone is the least dependable. Progesterone injections, because of their oil base, are painful and can cause sterile abscesses.

4. You must use progesterone during the symptomatic phase of the cycle—that is, from some time around ovulation until menstruation. It works best if started just before symptoms begin each month, but if you start too early, ovulation is stopped and irregular spotting or bleeding may follow.

5. Continue taking the progesterone until bleeding (not spotting) occurs. If you stop before then, you may have a rebound effect or crash, with worse PMS symptoms than before treatment. Sometimes you need to take the progesterone for a couple of days after bleeding begins in order to prevent this crash. PMS symptoms can also return several days after progesterone is stopped, so that the PMS symptoms now occur early in the cycle instead of premenstrually. Count the first day of your cycle as the day you *bleed,* not the day you begin spotting.

6. Women who have a very short symptom-free time each month may find themselves taking progesterone all month. Since the hormone works best if administered before symptoms occur and may need to be

continued after bleeding begins, the time span without medication may become shorter and shorter. The major difficulty with constant progesterone use is frequent spotting and bleeding.

7. If large doses of progesterone are being used rectally and are not effective, stool in the rectum may be preventing absorption. Timing dosage so the medication can be administered after a bowel movement can be beneficial, as can using a glycerin suppository to empty the bowel before inserting the progesterone. Since using laxatives or suppositories on a regular basis is never a good idea, this should be tried only in extreme situations.

8. If you are taking too much or absorbing too much progesterone, you may have sleepiness, confusion, and lethargy.

9. Progesterone is usually taken early in the morning and then sometimes again in the afternoon. When progesterone was first used in the United States, the manufacturer warned about insomnia as a potential side effect. This has not been the case, and many women take progesterone at night in order to ease their early-morning hours.

> *I take it at bedtime so I won't clench my teeth in my sleep. My dentist has noticed an improvement already.*

10. Women with PMS who have had hysterectomies may need to take progesterone throughout the month if their symptoms cannot easily be predicted by dates.

11. You can stop progesterone at the end of any cycle. It does not take several months to go off the substance. Just stop it at menstruation and don't start again. If your PMS varies from month to month, you can take it just during your difficult cycles.

12. You may be able to discontinue progesterone treatment after a year or two and not need it at all, or only for occasional cycles. On the other hand, you may need to take it for many years. Experience with progesterone and PMS is new in the United States, but we are beginning to see women successfully go off the hormone after two or three years of treatment. There is no way to know this in advance. PMS may disappear with menopause or it may continue as a cyclic problem even without menses.

13. The usual dosage in the United States ranges from 200 to 4,000 milligrams—this is not a typographical error; the range is that great—daily in one or several doses. Cost of progesterone therapy can run between $15 and $200 per month depending on the dose and source of the progesterone.

14. Progesterone rarely works for women with premenstrual magnification (PMM).

15. Minute doses of progesterone given just under the skin is now being tried on the theory that PMS is an allergy to one's own progesterone. The injections are given to desensitize the body. Some women have responded to this treatment, but it is still too early to tell its ultimate usefulness.

Side Effects

Undesirable side effects from progesterone are not usual, but when they do occur, irregular spotting and bleeding are most common, followed by diarrhea and cramping. The most severe but rare side effect has been hemorrhaging lasting about ten days.

POSSIBLE SIDE EFFECTS FROM RECTAL AND VAGINAL PREPARATIONS: breast tenderness, delayed menses, early menses, prolonged and irregular spotting, increased menstrual cramps, heavier or lighter periods, shorter or longer cycles, gas, weight gain, decreased sexual drive, faintness, headaches, allergic skin reaction, vaginal yeast infections.

POSSIBLE SIDE EFFECTS FROM INJECTABLE PREPARATIONS: All of the above but with the added potential of sterile abscesses at the site of injection. Injections are painful, as are the abscesses. However, for women who do not seem to be absorbing progesterone rectally, vaginally, or sublingually, this may be worth trying.

POSSIBLE SIDE EFFECTS FROM SUBLINGUAL PREPARATIONS: Same as rectal and vaginal, but added potential for faintness, especially after any alcohol or any period of fasting. Absorption is very uneven and some women do not respond to it at all. You should already be established on progesterone therapy before trying this method so that its actions can be more easily assessed.

ADDICTION: It is not clear whether progesterone is acting as a replacement hormone, much in the way insulin does for diabetes, or as a drug, as aspirin does for pain or inflammation. If we use the model of insulin, then being on progesterone constantly doesn't constitute an addiction any more than taking insulin does. However, if it is acting as a therapeutic agent, as aspirin, or as Valium, then needing it throughout the month does constitute an addictive process. In the absence of an answer to this question, we need simply to recognize the questions raised and the potential for having to use progesterone continuously. This problem has occurred most in women who have a very short symptom-free time, and in women with PMM. Often the progesterone has only slightly alleviated the problem of PMM, but the woman has then had difficulty discontinuing the medication at the end of each cycle.

Although progesterone has been used in England to treat PMS since 1948, there are no long-term controlled studies of its safety in humans. There are, however, some studies indicating that progesterone increases the risk of breast tumors in animals prone to develop tumors. To add to the confusion about safety, some progestogens are used to *treat* cancer. And there is some evidence that women with breast cancer have a lower progesterone level than normal, so it is conceivable that for those women, progesterone therapy could have a protective effect. Until large numbers of women have been studied over many years, the question of safety will remain unanswered. As with any treatment, a woman must weigh the risks of the treatment vs. the severity of the problem and then make as informed a decision as possible.

Progesterone, although not FDA approved for this purpose, is also currently being used to treat luteal phase defect. This is a newly recognized condition in which it is believed that insufficient progesterone levels cause infertility and very early spontaneous abortions (miscarriages in the first four to eight weeks of pregnancy). Progesterone suppositories in much lower dosages (25 to 50 milligrams per day) than what is common for PMS are being used. There are no controlled long-term studies demonstrating its safety, but it is being given in the belief that there are no dangers to its use. Unlike progesterone, *progestogens* have been found to cause an increase in birth defects following fetal exposure to those substances.

If you are planning to become pregnant, you should not take progesterone during the cycles in which you plan to conceive. Dr. Dalton has given progesterone to women throughout their pregnancies with no evident deleterious effects on the offspring. However, in the absence of large controlled studies, it is safest to discontinue the medication if you discover that you are pregnant. Progesterone is almost entirely excreted by the body within a day of taking it, so there is no need to stop the medication several cycles before you plan to become pregnant.

The FDA has not approved of the use of progesterone for PMS, but it has approved it for other uses. However, the FDA has not approved of any of the following drugs for PMS even though they are widely used for treatment of PMS:

TRANQUILIZERS: Valium, Miltown, Compazine, Xanax, etc.
DIURETICS: Hydrodiuril, Triamterene, Spironolactone, etc.
ANTIDEPRESSANTS: Elavil, Triavil, Parnate, Tofranil, etc.
HORMONES: Oral contraceptives, Provera, Depo-Provera, etc.
DIET PILLS AND STIMULANTS
SLEEPING PILLS

Hysterectomy and electroshock therapy do not fall within the bounds of FDA approval or disapproval, but both are dangerous and unproven treatments being used for PMS.

Studies

Other than reports by women and physicians that progesterone is helpful for PMS, it is difficult to evaluate the effectiveness of this treatment. The following problems exist with the research:

- No uniform definition exists of what constitutes PMS.
- Treatment schedules have varied from study to study.
- Results by one researcher have not been reproducible by the next.

The most useful studies are usually what are called double-blind studies in which neither the patient nor the practitioner knows whether she is getting a drug or a placebo, an inert drug made to look like the one being studied. However, women with the most severe forms of PMS usually object to being in such studies because, understandably, they want to be sure they get the progesterone, not the placebo. Therefore, those women who *do* enroll in such a study usually have less severe PMS, so the results become less applicable to women with severe illness.

All the studies of PMS, whether of progesterone, diuretics, or antidepressants have shown that even the placebo has the effect of improving PMS.

Conclusions?

Progesterone has been effective for many women in relieving their premenstrual symptoms. Percentages and efficacy rates are not clear. Long-terms effects are not clear. Difficult as it may be, women with PMS cannot for the present time expect to have clear, reassuring answers but must weigh their own difficulties and fears in deciding how their PMS will be treated.

Some women worry more about potential long-term problems. Others feel so incapacitated by their symptoms that immediate relief is more important to them than any potential long-term consequences. And others, playing both sides of the dilemma, decide to try a treatment but assume they will escape whatever long-term effects there might be.

If you are seeking treatment for PMS and considering progesterone therapy, read all you can, consider your fears, take them seriously, and try to choose within the context of your present life. Recognize too that decisions about treatment can be changed at any time. At this time there isn't a yes/no answer that applies to everyone because there is too little information and few certainties.

Women come for help with their PMS at various times in their cycles. When women are premenstrual they often have difficulty articulating their problems and making choices about treatment. Often they just want it to go away, regardless of any risk. When they are not premenstrual they are better able to weigh alternatives, but they also tend to underestimate how terrible they will feel premenstrually and will often decide not to use medication. Sometimes a week or so after a consultation, the woman will call saying, "It's worse than I thought and I want to try the progesterone." Some women who initially come for progesterone and decide to use it will decide by their next cycle that they want to try diet and exercise first. Flexibility, patience with the process of treatment, and compassion for oneself are the most important elements in designing your course of treatment.

CHAPTER 13

⊠

Antiprostaglandins, Antidepressants, and Diuretics

PROSTAGLANDINS ARE A GROUP OF HORMONES that help to regulate the contractions of muscles in some internal organs. One theory about PMS holds that an excess of these chemicals is being secreted in the woman suffering from PMS and therefore there are excessive contractions of the uterus, gastrointestinal tract, blood vessels, etc. Prostaglandins may also be involved in stress reactions and thereby directly influence the hypothalamus. (To continue the confusion as to etiology of PMS, the oil of evening primrose discussed in Chapter 11 is given in the belief that there is a *deficiency* of one of the prostaglandins.)

Antiprostaglandins are a group of drugs related to aspirin that have been used for years to treat arthritis. More recently they have also been found helpful for dysmenorrhea, or severe menstrual cramps. Such premenstrual physical symptoms as cramps, headaches, bloating, nausea, or breast pain are also sometimes responsive to antiprostaglandin medications. Some of the more common drugs with antiprostaglandin activity are aspirin, Motrin, Ponstel, Naprosyn, Anaprox, and Indocin. As with other drugs, the FDA has not approved antiprostaglandins for use in PMS.

Antiprostaglandins are administered orally, as pills, during the time of symptoms. The most common side effects are gastrointestinal irritation, with nausea, gas, or diarrhea.

Antidepressants

> *I have been hospitalized for depression three times in*
> *the past ten years. After the first time I was put on Elavil.*
> *Since then I have used every antidepressant they could find,*
> *including lithium. None of them worked. The fact that I*
> *was depressed only premenstrually was not discovered until*
> *two years ago. I had started charting on my own just to*
> *see when it was happening and found it was always near*
> *my period.*

Antidepressant therapy is not particularly effective for treating the depression of PMS, although it can at times lessen the general level of depression, leaving only a core of premenstrual symptoms that then become more noticeable.

Following is a list of the various types of antidepressants:

TRICYCLICS AND RELATED COMPOUNDS: There are many tricyclic antidepressants which are widely used—Aventyl, Elavil, Tofranil, Norpramin, Sinequan, and Vivactil, to name a few. All of these drugs are somewhat sedating. Other major side effects are constipation, dry mouth, blurred vision, gastrointestinal difficulties, heart palpitations and irregularities, difficulty reaching orgasm, weight gain, urinary retention, and orthostatic hypotension (where getting up suddenly produces a drop in blood pressure and subsequent faintness). There are also rare but possible serious long-term effects from taking such drugs regularly. These include blood disorders, jaundice, and heart difficulties. Antidepressants tend to interact with other medications, so you should always check with a doctor before *combining* antidepressant therapy with any other medications. All antidepressants work only when they reach a certain blood level over a period of time. Therefore results are not seen in less than two to three weeks. And upon discontinuation (which should never be abrupt and which should be with medical consultation), the effects of stopping are not known for two to three weeks.

MAO INHIBITORS: Parnate, Nardil, and Marplan are some of the most commonly prescribed MAO inhibitors. These drugs are considered stronger antidepressants than tricyclics and have some potentially serious side effects. Their use must be weighed carefully. In addition, they have the same general side effects as the tricyclics and in rare cases can produce agitation, confusion, and hallucinations. They are much more strongly reactive with other medications and with certain foods. Taking a MAO inhibitor involves being on a very strict diet from which many common and nutritious foods such as cheeses, chicken liver, yeast, and citrus fruits must be omitted.

LITHIUM SALTS: This medication, which has been in and out of favor over the years, is currently used for manic-depressive illness. While it appears quite effective in controlling the excitable (manic) phase of the manic-depressive cycle, it requires frequent monitoring of the patient's blood to protect against possible adverse changes in blood chemistry. In general, it is not prescribed for depression alone without careful consideration of its side effects, particularly since its effectiveness for depression is still controversial. While both manic-depressive illness and PMS are cyclic, it is PMS that is tied to the menstrual cycle.

To date, no one antidepressant has been found to be more effective than another for the depression of PMM. The FDA has not approved of any of the antidepressants for premenstrual syndrome.

Diuretics

Diuretics (water pills) have been widely used for PMS, though they have had little success in alleviating most of the symptoms. While they do remove fluid from the body, they can also cause an increase in lethargy and in feeling generally awful. They can cause excessive fluid loss and dehydration. For women trying to lose weight, this fluid loss can result in confusion and unhappiness, since they often erroneously believe they have lost fat weight rather than water. The frequent combination of diuretic and laxative abuse results in women living in a constantly dehydrated and electrolyte-depleted state.

Spironolactone, a widely used diuretic with some antidepressant qualities, is at times effective for PMS. Unfortunately, it stimulates tumor growth in rats.

Herbal diuretics are sometimes successful in relieving the bloated feeling. For example, raspberry leaf tea, made with dried raspberry leaves (1 teaspoon of leaves steeped in 1 cup water) or teas made from parsley, thyme, and chamomile may be useful for some women. Cucumber, corn silk, (excellent chopped up in salad) and watermelon are also mildly diuretic.

As we have discussed, simply drinking plain water may actually reduce bloating.

CHAPTER 14

⊠

Acupuncture and Other Alternative Therapies

Acupuncture

Eastern medicine views the mind and body as closely related and as made up of energy flows. PMS is thus seen by acupuncturists as an imbalance in the body's vital energy. Diagnosis involves determining whether the problem is one of excess energy, energy deficiency, or an energy blockage, and then knowing where, along the paths of energy flow, the imbalance is located. Fine needles are used to stimulate specific acupuncture points so that the flow of energy is regulated and blockages are removed. As with other treatments, it is not clear when acupuncture will or will not work. When successful, treatment may last for several months, with periodic "tune-ups" to maintain a balanced state.

As with all other treatments for PMS, there are practitioners and patients who claim that this is the one treatment that works. And for some it well may be. Women have sought acupuncture treatment before medical treatment, believing that it is more natural and safe. However, some have become worse before they have gotten better with acupuncture. Others have obtained relief more immediately, and still others have gone on for many months with little improvement.

Currently some work is being done to investigate the biochemical effects of acupuncture. There is speculation that acupuncture affects neurotransmitter levels, which as described earlier has direct effects on the hypothalamus.

Chiropractic Adjustment

Many women have been relieved of their premenstrual symptoms after chiropractic treatments. Chiropractic is based on the principle that the entire body is affected by the spine; appropriate adjustment of the spine can therefore alleviate dysfunctioning systems. This method is not well accepted within the medical community, but has in fact offered considerable relief to many with PMS.

Acupressure, foot reflexology, therapeutic massage, and therapeutic touch are all systems of working with body energy to effect change. While they are only recently becoming widely used and accepted in Western medicine, they are all methods of healing that have been developed and used by other cultures for centuries. Although obviously you can apply pressure to your own foot or chest or other parts of the body, these techniques usually work best if someone else does them to/for you. In all healing there is the aspect of the healer and what that person brings to the method in terms of his/her own energy, desire to help, and technical skills.

The following methods of healing, as well as many others not described here, have at times been beneficial in reducing the immediate tension and stress of PMS. There are books about each of these techniques. Some of them are simple enough for you to learn with a partner so you can help each other. If you are going to use any of these methods, you must be prepared for the emotions that may be freed and expressed as a result of therapy. Working on the body often results in a surfacing of repressed feelings. Their expression may also be beneficial to you, but in any event, do not be surprised by their sometimes unexpected appearance.

Acupressure

Acupressure is similar to acupuncture but is conducted without needles. Pressure is applied to particular points on the body in order to change the flow of energy. Usually the points to be used are identified both by their location on body maps and by the pain produced when pressure is applied. However, even a light touch can give you some relief from symptoms.

Foot Reflexology

This unique method relies on identified points on the foot that correspond to both internal and external parts of the body. Special points are said to balance hormones. Foot reflexology can be relaxing and soothing for the entire body. Especially if you are somewhat anxious about having your body worked on, this is an extremely effective and nonthreatening way to introduce yourself to these methods. Foot reflexology requires removing only your socks or stockings. Results can feel quite similar to having had a total body massage.

Therapeutic Massage

I use this term to include several massage techniques. Various forms of massage are designed to effect deeper changes in the body tension level. Some are vigorous and others are quite gentle. Some can be done while you remain entirely clothed, while others require more direct access to your skin surface. Some of the gentler forms of massage allow for greater relaxation and deeper responses (this author's preference).

Therapeutic Touch

This is a recently developed system derived from ancient healing principles. It is widely practiced by nurses and other health professionals. The practitioner works on the energy field around a person rather than directly on the body. It is done while you are fully clothed, simply sitting in a straight-backed chair. Energy is both felt and directed by the practitioner in order to give relief from symptoms.

Some of you may find these methods and even the language in which they are described to be quite strange. Others may be both surprised and relieved to see them described as healing modalities. PMS stretches us to grow. Its complexity, its pervasiveness, and its persistence often push us to search beyond culturally accepted procedures. For many women with PMS, treatment is a journey that motivates them to take risks in sharing their PMS experiences, in trying various kinds of treatment programs, and in looking for answers beyond those offered by traditional Western medicine.

CHAPTER 15

⬚

Psychotherapy

Some women suffering from PMS have been helped and others hurt by traditional psychotherapy, depending on the views of the specific psychotherapist toward premenstrual tension and women's problems in general. Without a recognition of the biological component in premenstrual symptoms, the woman is made to feel that the changes she experiences are a result of psychopathology and that she ought to be able to prevent them. In fact the specific *emotional* symptoms that a woman manifests premenstrually may be related to her particular personality, strengths, weaknesses, strivings, history, and drives. But the mood swings and the cyclic physiological changes are more a matter of her biological makeup.

Psychotherapy can be beneficial in helping a woman explore the specific emotional issues that upset her premenstrually. Whatever a woman is suppressing or trying to forget is likely to surface when she is premenstrual. Acknowledging and dealing with emotions usually bottled up or denied make them less likely to become overwhelming premenstrually.

We live in a society in which women are not encouraged to express anger, aggression, or ambition. It is often in the protection of a therapeutic relationship, therefore, that women first become able to express their anger and their suppressed needs. Most women find it difficult to allow themselves comfort and pleasure. It often requires another person, a friend or a therapist, to help a woman begin to nurture and care for herself, to experience the self-love that is essential for well-being.

There are therefore real benefits to be gained from psychotherapy for the woman with PMS, providing the therapist and the client recognize the full complexity of premenstrual changes and the interplay of body, mind, and emotion. The therapy must be directed at the integration of all these factors.

CHAPTER 16

⊠

Support Groups

The object is to break the silence and to know that you are not alone.

Doctor, when you told me there had been other women whose PMS did not respond to any treatment, I suddenly didn't feel so alone anymore. I thought, there are others like me.

Consciousness-raising groups in the sixties and seventies helped many women validate their own experiences as women. Today PMS support groups, which have already begun to form in many communities, serve the same function. Many women have believed that they were the only ones with premenstrual difficulties, have felt helpless to do anything about them, or have been ashamed to reveal the extent of their difficulties. These groups provide a place where women can begin to share their concerns. They also provide a support network of women on whom to call when depressed, overwhelmed, or uncontrollably angry.

The following are some guidelines for starting and running such groups:

1. Place an ad in a local paper or try posting notices at some of the following places: supermarket bulletin boards, work bulletin boards (depending on how safe that feels), Y's, health clubs, churches.

2. Meet in each other's homes, Y's, churches, schools, day-care centers or nursery schools.

3. Set an initial time period—for instance, two or three months—during which you can meet, and then reevaluate whether the group is helpful.

4. Rotate leadership, with everyone taking a turn, or else each of a core group of originators.

5. Don't be afraid to close membership for a period of time so that you can get to know one another. You might leave membership open for a month and then close it. There is always a conflict between being open for new members who may need the group but who also create some disruption, and getting to know and trust a stable group of women. Even if you do close the group you always have the option of reopening it for new people.

6. Remember that it's not just PMS problems that come to a group, but *women* with PMS as well as other social and medical problems that may or may not be related to the PMS. Don't try to cure everyone of everything.

7. Collect money for any expenses so that no one person feels burdened.

8. Make a challenge of providing refreshments that are compatible with PMS dietary guidelines. (Don't forget popcorn!)

9. Create telephone trees for contacting people, both to create a support network and to ensure that the burden of the group does not fall on one or two people.

10. Rotate responsibilities regarding phone calls from/to new people seeking help or information.

11. Structure how women will speak. For instance, allow each person to speak for a set time with no interruptions and be sure every woman gets to talk without interruption before discussion is thrown open to everyone.

12. Structure the time. If a meeting is to be three hours, allow time for "war stories" of suffering and past treatment difficulties and then go on to an agenda. This allows people a chance both to vent feelings and then

to be involved in some constructive planning and support. Use the contents page of this or any other book about PMS as a guideline for each week.

13. You may want to learn some alternative healing methods together so you can help each other during difficult times. For instance, some or all of you can attend massage or foot reflexology workshops, or you may be able to have a practitioner give a workshop for the whole group.

14. Try role-playing of premenstrual personalities. This is difficult at first, but as you begin to share your "monsters" they lose some of their frightening and controlling aspects.

15. Don't forget humor. In the worst of it all, the ability to laugh at oneself can be life-saving.

Support groups can occasionally generate stress or trauma. Some of the PMS groups have ended with disappointment or bitterness. While this can happen with any group, there are some particular problems and pitfalls for women starting and belonging to PMS groups.

• Coming to define one's life by PMS. There is/was more to life than PMS, but it is easy, especially when you are experiencing enthusiasm of validation, for life to become centered around PMS. Some women will decide to devote a great deal of time to PMS, but that should be a conscious decision, not a situation you just fall into.
• Burnout from trying to take care of all the needs of others. Learning to help and also to say no is always a challenge.
• The belief that one's own PMS has to be cured in order to be helpful to others. The persistence of PMS symptoms has to be understood by everyone because the group will have to deal with all the tensions and mood swings characteristic of PMS. It doesn't necessarily go away because you are a leader or a member of a PMS group.
• It's easy to become angry that someone has PMS and is behaving in a disruptive way. In a way, the PMS group gives women a chance to experience what those around them do on a regular basis when they are suffering from PMS.
• Competition over whose PMS is worst and who has the worst horror stories.

Support groups will not cure PMS, but they can make it more manageable. One of the most devastating aspects of any illness is the isolation it can create.

There is no way to underestimate how important it is in our society, where people move a great deal, leave familiar places, friends, and families, to be in a group with others "like me."

PART III

Broader Aspects of PMS

CHAPTER 17

Sexuality and PMS

Margaret

Margaret lay in bed staring at the ceiling. Restless, she tried not to move, aware of Kurt on the other side of the bed. They lay facing away from each other, the strain of their fighting showing in the distance between them in the bed. She knew he'd be asleep soon and the long night would be hers alone.

Maybe, if her sleep were quiet she too would be able to rest. But instead of rest she had nightmares in which she kept losing control. The most recent ones had been of cars. Some she was driving, some Kurt or an unrecognizable stranger, but in each dream the car would eventually go out of control. She had driven off mountains and along the ocean floor (in that one some air masks had mysteriously appeared as the car sank deeper into the water), and last night a long-forgotten teacher from third grade appeared in time to keep her car from swerving off into a gravel pit.

A part of her wished she could lean over and touch Kurt's body, feel the warmth that at times made all her other fears disappear. What if she did move closer? What was the penalty of reaching across? Would the anger she expressed at him come back at her? She wasn't proud of the words she had spoken. She knew her last spate of accusations had hit him deeply. She listened to his breathing, guessing that he was still awake but that he wanted her to believe he was asleep. It was another piece of his escape. If she moved over, if she touched him, would he also think she was taking back everything she had said?

Self-contained—that's how she usually thought of herself, but tonight the restlessness in her body made her want to fling herself away from her confusion, her unexpected fears, anger, tears. . . . I'm self-contained and self-sufficient, she thought, except lately I haven't been that way very much.

Sometimes she imagined that her anger at Kurt came from knowing that she could not reach across to ask him to hold her. Before she could even express her needs to him, she was angry for his presumed refusal. And, what if he thought she wanted to make love? How could she tell him she wanted only to be held? Sex is a mystery, and years of marriage, books, and talking had not make it any clearer. Recently she hadn't wanted to make love a lot of the time and that had put its own strain on their relationship. Doing it when she didn't want to was terrible. Tonight she wanted to be held and didn't want sex. Kurt usually had trouble with that. He'd get angry and then they'd be fighting again.

Margaret doesn't have to have PMS to be in her current situation. In fact hers is not an uncommon experience for women in our culture. The issues raised here regarding sexuality are relevant to women with PMS and without it. The importance, however, of PMS to sexuality is that most women with PMS do experience some change in their sex drive premenstrually. Some have a greatly increased sex drive, while others lose theirs altogether. Depression is usually associated with a decreased libido, but in PMS there is not always a clear association. A woman can be premenstrually depressed and withdrawn and still have an increased sex drive, although the opposite is more common.

Premenstrually some women also find that their body changes in ways affecting their sexuality. Breast tenderness can be so severe as to make any touching of the nipples painful. Bloating can make a woman feel both uncomfortable and unattractive.

Body size is often as much as a matter of fashion as of health. There is a story told of an anthropologist visiting an African tribe, and seeing a young woman dramatically tugging hard at her firm breasts. When queried, she explained that she was trying to make them hang the way a grown woman's is supposed to, which in that culture was a sign of maturity. Without our own cultural bias toward thinness, premenstrual women might even be able to boast about their cyclicly protruding abdomens. Women, of course, say that they feel better when they are not bloated, but some of that sense of well-being comes from seeing ourselves through other people's eyes. Nothing kills libido or self-esteem quite like feeling ugly.

Sensuality, the need to touch and be touched, to hold and be held, must be differentiated from genital sexuality. Many women have an increased need for intimacy premenstrually while at the same time being either neutral or repelled by sexuality. This can be confusing to the woman as well as to her partner, who may interpret the overtures toward intimacy as requests for sexuality.

Sexuality cannot be separated from the people engaged in a sexual or potentially sexual relationship. All the dynamics of PMS which play themselves out in other areas will also exist within the realm of sexuality. How a woman feels about herself and her sexuality will play a part in how her premenstrual sexual changes are expressed. A woman who is in a celibate relationship will experience an increased libido premenstrually differently from one who is sexually active in a relationship. The change in her drive will have different meanings and consequences for both her and her partner.

For instance, a woman with an increased sex drive premenstrually can seek out her partner and express her sexual needs. She can seek out new partners. She can masturbate. She can remain sexually stimulated and take no action toward having those needs met.

Which option a woman chooses will depend on how she feels about her sexuality, whether she is in a primary relationship, how she feels about touching herself and masturbating, and so forth. And at different times in her life she may choose differently.

For women with decreased libido, the issues are slightly different and more often depend on what is happening in an ongoing sexual relationship. For instance:

• To what extent does she feel she has a choice about when she has sexual relations?

- Is her lack of desire premenstrually specific to one partner?
- Is her desire marginal anyway and simply absent premenstrually?
- Is she free to express her needs for affection without sexuality, and is her partner receptive to those needs?
- Is the lack of sexual desire connected to an increase in psychological vulnerability?
- Are there sexual conflicts in the non-premenstrual time?
- Can she separate out issues of premenstrual irritability, anxiety, anger, depression, from sexual needs?

A Sexual Inventory

Looking at your own views about sexuality can be helpful in understanding and coping with premenstrual sexual changes. The following questions are meant to stimulate thought on the subject. They are not questions with right or wrong answers, but are intended to help simplify what is often seen as an entanglement of sexuality.

1. What are your basic beliefs about sexuality?

2. What are your feelings about touching yourself, sexual play, masturbation, or making love to yourself? It is amazing how many women have read or heard enough to believe that it is normal for children to masturbate but have not been able to believe that this is also true for themselves.

3. Have your sexual experiences been gratifying for you? Have you experienced orgasm? With a partner? By yourself?

4. Have you ever found yourself using sex as a favor or withholding it as a punishment?

5. What are your feelings about initiating of sexual activity?

6. Do you feel you can refuse to have sex?

7. What are your religious beliefs about sex?

8. Are you afraid of your partner?

9. Is your partner afraid of you?

10. The assumption is that we are all modern and liberated these days, but what are your feelings about sex in relation to shame, guilt, pleasure, sin, and punishment?

11. Do you feel free to talk about sexuality with your partner or partners when you have them? Another anomaly of our culture is that many people will easily take off their clothes and have sex with someone else but will not feel free to talk with him or her about it.

12. Do you feel free to express what you like/dislike in sexuality?

13. Do you feel your partner has the right to say no? Do you get angry? Do you feel hurt?

14. How are your feelings about sexuality related to your feelings about your body? For example, do you think of your sexuality as being related to your weight or fitness?

Take some time to look over this inventory. Many of these questions may take a long time to answer, and you may have different answers for them at different times in your life. Keep in mind both your general answers and how they may vary during the menstrual cycle. For instance, you may feel comfortable about initiating sexual activity, but premenstrually you may *need* your partner to take more initiative. Or you may think of yourself as someone who enjoys her sexuality, but premenstrually you just don't want to be touched at all.

Sexuality and PMS Treatment

Treatment for PMS may or may not affect sexual aspects of the cyclic changes. Obviously if women are less depressed, less angry, and less anxious, their sexual responses will be more directly connected to their feelings about sexuality and their relationships. As couples begin to develop ways of communicating about PMS and sexuality changes, they also will be able to be more responsive to each other. Compromise and communication by both partners can obviously lead to more satisfying relationships.

One of the more common dynamics of a couple is for the woman with PMS to withdraw sexually premenstrually and for her partner to be threatened by this withdrawal and to want sexual relations even more. Often the more one person pulls away, the more the other is in pursuit. Even if a couple is having sexual relations once a week, for example, the withdrawal may leave the other partner wanting it daily, as reassurance that the relationship and its sexual component are intact. Treatment of PMS along with explanations of dynamics such as these often helps a couple to get through the premenstrual period with their relationship intact, even if there is no actual change in the frequency of sexual contact.

Problems of decreased libido have to date been the PMS symptoms least responsive to therapy, and this holds true even for the medical treatments. Progesterone for some women causes a decrease in sexual drive even if there hadn't been a pronounced cyclic depression in that drive previously.

Problems of increased sex drive have been somewhat easier to deal with, since these tend to be less threatening to most relationships. The changes in sexuality associated with PMS are not a problem per se unless the woman and her partner view them as such.

CHAPTER 18

✶

The Family and PMS

He asked how he could help and I said, "Love me through it."

PMS affects women, and when women are part of a family, it affects the family. When a mother has PMS, when a teenage daughter has PMS, when a grandmother has PMS, the entire family group may be affected.

Women differ as to who receives the brunt of their PMS. Some women turn it inwards and become depressed or suicidal; others turn on partners, children, or colleagues at work. The inconsistency and unpredictability of mood swings are usually the most difficult aspects of PMS for the woman and others. Remember, though, everyone has moods, needs, problems, anger and conflicts in relationships.

While there are some women whose PMS simply goes away with treatment, many other women and their families must continue to grapple with some cyclic mood swings. In certain families there may be a residue of emotions that continue to affect everyone even after the PMS itself is under control. And in still others, the PMS was never really the major problem and its resolution has made more obvious the ways in which the family is in difficulty.

Husbands and PMS

Men do not get PMS, but when they are close to a woman with PMS, they become involved in the dynamics of the problems. Men don't make PMS happen, but at times their own personality traits contribute to the premenstrual discord. In our society, women tend to be more emotional, or at least more expressive of their emotions, and are even more openly emotional premenstrually. Thus a relationship already strained by a discrepancy in expressiveness will be even more strained when the woman is premenstrual. Most of the women I have talked with, both with and without PMS, have described their husbands or boyfriends as rarely talking about personal problems, not being emotional, "keeping everything in," and often being angry at the woman's needs for expression.

Silas, in the following anecdote, is like many men I have seen with their wives, men who have come to talk about their wives or lovers, and men who have been described to me by unhappy and at times lonely women. In comparison with most of these men, he is neither the most macho nor the most sensitive. And like most of them, Silas is indeed trying his best.

Silas

Silas slouched in the crushed velvet armchair of Dr. Adaire's office and stared silently at the slightly off-center portrait on the far wall. Therapy was a concession to his wife and their marriage counselor. He didn't want to be here, but he was willing to give it a try. He wanted to make their lives together better, but this office, the words spoken here, were foreign to him.

"Women are the emotional center of the family." That's what had been said several sessions before, and Silas had no disagreement with that statement. Mothers were emotional. His mother had been, his wife was. His father hadn't been and neither was he. In spite of all the recent propaganda telling boys it was okay to cry, Silas found a certain comfort in the old order, in a clarity that defined men's and women's needs and their expressions differently. Why change it? Why change anything?

Sure, sometimes life had its pains, but you kept a stiff upper lip and went on.

But each month, before Elizabeth, his wife, got her period, the lid was loosened off a caldron of resentments. She'd say something cutting and suddenly Silas's face would flush, his arms and chest become tight, and he'd have to sit very still so that he wouldn't explode. Even as he thought about it, he could feel his body tensing. Her emotions frightened him.

Listening to Dr. Adaire, Silas was reluctant to engage in the difficult task of communicating. He remembered being three years old and seeing words on a page. At the time he couldn't imagine how those symbols would ever take meaningful form for him. Once he'd learned to read, though, it was odd remembering not being able to read. He wondered if that would ever be true for this experience.

He forced his attention back to the room, to Dr. Adaire, and to what he was supposed to be doing here. He was supposed to talk, and then somehow their marriage was supposed to get better. Still, there was something good about getting it off his chest, even if it didn't change anything. Women expressed their feelings and men got it off their chests.

"I can't seem to make her happy," Silas said. "At that time of the month, everything I do is wrong."

Silas's wife has PMS, and they as a couple have difficulties. Even without PMS, there are times when they will be in conflict. Silas will feel confused, as if something were being asked of him that he can't understand. Elizabeth will feel isolated because he can't seem to hear what she is saying or be sympathetic to her feelings.

The belief that all will be well when a woman's PMS is treated is a fantasy that assigns all the family's troubles to the woman and her PMS. Unfortunately, treatment may not only leave areas of conflict unresolved but may even accentuate other problems in the relationship.

> *He hits me when I'm premenstrual. I know I provoke*
> *him, but every time it happens, I'm still surprised. I feel*
> *so bad about myself, I think I must have deserved this.*

Then after my period I get angry with myself for letting
him do that to me and for staying with him.

Sometimes the woman with PMS seems to express emotions for both herself and her partner. Although dreaded, the explosions become an emotional purge for everyone involved. In a marriage, the woman's anger often becomes an excuse for the man to let go of his. When the woman gains more control over her emotions and this dynamic changes, the couple is left without this outlet and must begin to develop new ways of releasing tension, both individually and/or together.

When I have PMS, we all have PMS.

In a family with identified PMS, the mother often takes on the responsibility for all the moods of everyone. When she isn't cool, calm, or collected, she is considered ill, while others may act out anger, irritability, and even violence in "response" to her illness.

On the other hand, women with PMS often have an uncanny ability to lash out at another person's most vulnerable areas. They can be most insensitive and destructive, often deeply regretting what they have said, but nonetheless leaving the other person devastated and confused.

PMS is not confined to women in heterosexual relationships. Lesbian women seeking treatment for PMS and their partners often describe their difficulties with the relationship in words identical to women with PMS and their male partners. The same premenstrual tensions, accusations, and withdrawal exist. When the couple's menstrual cycles become synchronous and therefore both women are premenstrual at approximately the same time, the tensions, strains, and potential for explosions are even greater. Women often like to believe that they are more understanding than men of another woman's suffering, but in a relationship they tend to be as frustrated, impatient, needy, and vulnerable as the male partners of women with PMS.

PMS has at times been used by women as an excuse for abuse. People in relationships cannot be expected to take it just because the behavior has a medical name. Painful things are said and done. Though you may be sympathetic to a woman's PMS, there is still a need to get some distance, to protect yourself from the behavioral effects of PMS, whether these are physical or emotional. Separation can at times be helpful.

Teens, Moods, and PMS

Adolescence in our culture is a serious challenge. It is a challenge for the girl/boy, and a challenge for families, schools, and the community. Moodiness and lack of predictability are the norm at this time.

PMS may start with menarche, the time of a girl's first menstrual period, or a year or two earlier than that. To differentiate the general mood swings of adolescence from premenstrual changes is difficult, if not impossible. Teenagers tend to be much less articulate about how they are feeling than older people, at least with adults. And they also tend to deny any connection between their moods and their cycles. That association seems to imply to them that the moods are less real or that their feelings are less valid.

The diary of "Carly" illustrates some of these conflicts:

Thursday night

Dear Diary,

You must think that all I ever feel is sad because that's when I write to you. That's not true, though. Sometimes I feel really happy, but I guess I only need to write to you when I'm unhappy.

Today I'm unhappy and yesterday I was unhappy. Sometimes there is a good reason, but other times I just feel unhappy and then I find reasons. Like if someone says something to me one day it can be okay, but on another day I get angry at them or angry at myself.

My face . . . Sometimes I think I'm ugly, that my hair is ugly, that I'm fat, my legs are too fat. A voice inside me just whines with all the things wrong with me.

At school today I was standing in the lunch line and I saw Evie and Tori having lunch together and I just felt left out. Suddenly my eyes got red and I thought I was going to cry right there. I got out a tissue and pretended

I had to sneeze and then I started coughing so my red eyes wouldn't show so much. This is stupid. Why should I care? They're both creeps anyway. Then I came home and started working on the report due in history and I couldn't concentrate. It's stupid anyway. Who cares about kings? Kings are creeps.

Today in English class I couldn't concentrate at all. I kept thinking about a poem I wanted to write. The teacher got mad at me because she saw me writing notes, and when she called on me I was off in space and couldn't remember which book we were supposed to be reading. She said she is calling my mother because I keep doing this . . . something about not living up to my potential, I think.

Next month I'll be fifteen. If I live to seventy-five that's one fifth of my lifetime gone already. I might not even live that long.

Tuesday Afternoon

Dear Diary,

Last night I pigged out on two Reese's marshmallow fudge sundaes and a bag of chocolate chip cookies. This morning my face looks horrible and I HATE myself and I HATE everyone else too.

I yelled at Evie in the locker room because her bag pushed my towel onto the floor. YUK . . . I told her I didn't ever want to be her friend again. The locker room is filthy. I hate getting undressed and dressed to go do stupid dances.

Thank God I can shut the door to this room and be alone. If anyone else says anything else to me I'll hit them. Why is it some days everything goes wrong?

Carly's mother would not do well to say, "Carly, maybe you are premenstrual."

Carly may or may not have PMS. She does have moods, as do most adolescents, female and male. Only by charting can we relate her moods to her menstrual period. And if they are related, there is still the question as to whether we should consider anything to be wrong with her. If her moods are troublesome to her, she may want to try altering her diet, exercising, etc. If her moods are troublesome only for her family, she still has to decide if she wants to try to change herself at all. It does not work for the family to try to change an adolescent's PMS, just as it does not work for a spouse to try to treat a woman's PMS.

The only exception is in the area of women who are retarded or mentally incompetent and unable to take care of themselves. In that event, support people may begin treatment regimens to try to affect cyclic disturbing behavior by using diet changes or medications. In general it just doesn't work to try to treat someone else's PMS. Even with medication, there needs to be active cooperation on the part of the woman with PMS in order to achieve any success.

Telling Children About PMS

> One day I cleaned out my daughter's closet, locked myself inside, and screamed into a pillow. Later my son asked me if I'd heard a strange sound in the house.

Babies, toddlers, and small children are confused by mood changes. As they get older, children are better able to understand the inconsistencies of a mother suffering from PMS. Eventually they are even able to consciously modify their own behavior in relation to a mother's needs at some times of the month.

> Pretend that sometimes Mommy is inside a balloon and she needs some quiet and needs for you all to be gentle with her.

> Some days of the month Mommy yells when chores aren't done and other days she just laughs and tells you to do them. Can you figure out which days those are, and would you like to write them down?

However, children have their own needs, including the need for emotional release. They often know when a request will bring a yes or when it will provoke irritation or anger. When irritable or moody themselves, they can be adept at both provoking adult explosions and becoming the target of those explosions.

> *Eventually the boys learned that there were certain times when I needed to be left alone. Sometimes it was just to take a bath without being interrupted.*

Living in a culture in which we try to give our children the best, we find it hard to come to terms with our own shortcomings as parents. Guilt becomes a major obstacle to sharing the facts about PMS with our children. We don't want our children to have a "sick" parent. When the illness is barely understood and the reality of it is often doubted, the problems are confounded. Children can become caught in marital conflict over PMS, and most often this is conflict reflecting and expressing their father's anger toward their mother.

Can women with PMS be good mothers? Of course they can, depending on the severity of their problems and their ability to deal with them. As repeatedly stated, PMS can be mild or severe. It can interfere in some areas of a woman's life and not in others. And it is treatable.

Both mothers and fathers have moods. Although one question might be "Is Mommy premenstrual?" another should be "What mood will Daddy be in when he comes home tonight?"

Points to Remember for Family and PMS

1. PMS affects the entire family.

2. All family members have moods.

3. Identifying PMS does not make all the problems go away.

4. Treatment of PMS may not make all the problems go away.

5. Family support is important in life-style and dietary changes.

6. Some family problems may be related to PMS and others not.

7. Family members can be both victims and instigators of premenstrual explosions.

8. Being premenstrual is not an illness. Having moods is not an illness. Having severe premenstrual symptoms is.

9. The woman with PMS has to be responsible for her treatment herself. Others can only support her.

CHAPTER 19

Creativity
and PMS

I feel receptive premenstrually, and more sensitive. I take everything in but I can't discriminate well. Then later I have to try to figure it all out.

I get scared I'll get lost in my work. I'm in a frenzy with it and then I get my period and I'm different again.

I get surges of energy premenstrually and suddenly want to clean, move furniture, or write. There are real highs and lows.

For me sexual energy and creative energy seem to come at the same time in my cycle. For a while I'm driven crazy by both but I get a lot done and then I menstruate and I feel normal again.

Women may have a lessening of boundaries, of control, and of rules during the premenstrual time. They seem to be directed more by what is occurring internally than externally. While this can obviously lead to difficulties in living, it can also stimulate creative expression. Along with the lessening of constraint, there is also a heightened sensitivity to sound, sight, and smell. Colors may take on a different hue.

The ability to put expression into form is not improved during the premenstrual time. In other words, a writer may write well premenstrually but edit well after her period. An artist said:

> *I do sketches when I am premenstrual. That's when*
> *I get my ideas, but I never start the full drawing then. I*
> *can't get the lines the way I want them. I see them, but*
> *I can't do it right on the paper.*

Defining or explaining creativity may not be any easier than explaining God. We watch as children are creative on the beach making sand castles. Musicians are creative playing their instruments. Women are creative knitting or crocheting. Artists are creative in their painting or sculpting. They are all drawing on inner images of how something is to take shape. In each case, the final form reflects both agreed-upon societal patterns as well as an individual imprint.

What we usually do not consider creative is replicating what has been done—tracing a drawing, constructing a building exactly the same as all the others, turning over a pail of sand and saying that it's a castle. So creativity includes some individuality and some variation from standard blueprints. Premenstrually women are more aware of inner visions and less attached to blueprints.

Creativity has been tied to suffering. Whether in fact this is true, it does appear that some people can use their pain creatively. To the extent that PMS alters consciousness and produces pain, it can at times be a catalyst for new growth and meaning.

> *I would never have wished for PMS, but as a result*
> *of my illness I have a new and deeper understanding of*
> *others' suffering. I'd had an easy life until PMS. I hope*
> *now to help others who are in pain.*

CHAPTER 20

⊠

Social and
Political
Implications

MEDICAL TRENDS APPEAR within a political context. They grow out of the presumptions and ethics of a particular period of time. The new discovery, in 1981, of an old problem appeared when women's struggles for equality were being heavily countered. PMS appeared as the ERA was being defeated. The relationship between premenstrual tension and hormones had of course been described in 1931 by Dr. Robert T. Frank. Dr. Katharina Dalton had been talking and writing about PMS since 1953. Until that point, however, the predominant pieces of advice given to women with PMS were: take Valium, take amphetamines, take a vacation, take a lover, try alcohol, stop complaining, have a baby, have a hysterectomy, get married (don't get married), it's all in your head, you want to be this way. When PMS *was* recognized by segments of the health care community, women were often told that it was the result of their denial of the feminine role, hypochondriasis, neurosis, or "thinking too much."

The arrival of PMS in the United States came not out of medical concern for women's health but rather on the heels of British court cases in which women pleaded that their violent actions were the result of their uncontrollable PMS. Headlines in U.S. newspapers linked PMS with violence. After all, headlines about bloating, tension, or headaches don't sell papers. However, once PMS arrived in the United

States, it caught the attention of millions of women who finally felt validated in their own experiences of cyclic physical and emotional disturbances. At the same time it created some conflict within groups struggling for equal opportunities for women. Many feared that the recognition of PMS would result in a political setback for women, who would be portrayed as undependable, out of control, and therefore unworthy of political office, well-paying jobs, or custody of their children.

Few women, however, actually lose control premenstrually. There is no scientific evidence linking women's biology with violence, although studies have linked male hormones with aggressive behavior. The vast majority of crimes are still committed by men, not by women. Men, like women, have moods, as any wife, secretary, or nurse can attest. And men, like women, have times of increased and decreased productivity.

A woman with severe PMS will be limited by her illness. One with mild mood changes will not. Think of PMS as being analogous to arthritis, which can range from a few stiff joints on awakening in the morning to a crippling and incapacitating disease. If you are looking for a tennis champion, you would not expect to train someone with severe arthritis. A woman with an occasional elbow pain might go on to the championship. One who is crippled obviously would not, but if her arthritis was cured, she might still win. We do not disqualify the human race from tennis because some people have arthritis, but some circles would exclude *all* women because some get severe PMS.

The particular mood expressions of PMS, like anger, must also be seen in the context of a society that discourages women's anger, ambition, and independence. Sometimes this discouragement is overt, and other times it is a matter of inner voices internalized by the woman herself. The husband of a woman who came for help described their problem as follows:

> *My wife is fine for two weeks out of the month. She's friendly and a good wife. The house is clean. Then she ovulates and suddenly she's not happy about her life. She wants a job. She wants to go back to school. Then her period comes and she is all right again.*

Another woman described:

> *I'm a happy person with a good life. I have a husband who is good to me and three healthy children. Then when I'm premenstrual these thoughts come into my head like "What is the meaning of my life?" I don't have room for them! I just want them to go away.*

PMS and Responsibility

The issue of responsibility and PMS is a confusing one: "Is it my PMS or is it me?"

Each woman experiences her PMS somewhat differently, has more or less anger or sadness or irritability. If one woman expresses her PMS as suicidal fantasy and another as homicidal, then these two women have in their personalities certain destructive energies directed either toward themselves or toward others. There is no evidence for one kind of PMS that makes a woman suicidal as opposed to another that makes her homicidal or creative or causes her to shoplift.

I first learned of hypnosis as a child. My friends and I would talk about this mysterious force that would make you do something you would never do on your own. Then as I got older I learned that hypnosis could not make you be or do something that was totally against who you were and what your values were. I am still not sure what the real truth is about that, but the situation is similar in PMS. For the most part, people do not do things counter to their values, even when they are suffering from PMS.

The antisocial behavior of PMS is probably more a matter of premenstrual magnification (PMM) than of PMS. The women in England who committed crimes had histories of prior and subsequent antisocial behavior. To say that the premenstrual state magnified these impulses is more correct than to say that PMS caused their behavior.

PMS does seem to lessen the control with which people restrain impulses, and it seems to lessen their ability to deal with disturbing inner images. But the particular means of expression seems distinctly individual. No one's Mr. Hyde is exactly like another's. We have all had nightmares or bad dreams. My nightmares and yours may have similar themes, but there are individual differences specific to who I am and who you are. If my dreams or fantasies begin to seep into waking reality and I begin to act as though they are real, is that me? The lessening of boundaries may be biological or emotional or spiritual. At what point am I considered to have lost control? When am I responsible for what I have done as a result of having those dreams come into reality?

The questions become even more confusing when they relate to law. Law is a system of dealing with rules for a society and may not have much to do with truth, morality, or biology. However the courts decide issues concerning PMS and women's responsibility for their actions, they still won't answer the question of whether women are or are not responsible. They will say only how the legal system decides to view PMS at a certain point in history.

Legally defining women as not responsible will add to undesirable stereotypes of women. This defense, as any, may also be exploited by women who are unwilling to take responsibility for their actions, in the same way that men can exploit similar laws governing sanity and responsibility.

The danger in holding women entirely responsible for their actions is that many women with PMS would interpret that decision as not taking seriously the degree of impairment they experience as a result of their PMS. And many women maintain that they are not responsible for their actions premenstrually.

The issue is an emotionally charged one. Like abortion, it combines aspects of personal behavior and beliefs with societal rules and definition. Both men and women have very strong feelings about PMS, and arguments are often based on those emotions. Court decisions will have little impact on such emotions.

As for the ultimate question of responsibility, no one can truly answer that. We have no uniform way of deciding responsibility at any one time for any person. If six psychiatrists are trying to determine if someone is responsible for a crime, most often three will see it one way and three the other. And even if six people agree, whether they be six psychiatrists or six people off the street, that only means that they agree, not that they have determined truth.

The question of responsibility is broader than PMS but is nevertheless relevant. If we see ourselves as products of unfortunate circumstances or bodily processes, does that relieve us of responsibility for our actions? If a person is abused as a child, is that person not responsible for his/her actions in abusing children as an adult? To hold someone responsible does not negate the circumstances that may have contributed to those actions, but may do a disservice to those who have survived the past or present hardships and have been able, often through great pain and struggle, to overcome the destructive patterns of behavior.

CHAPTER 21

Getting Help
for PMS

PMS is persistent, and even with self-help solutions it may not go away or it may recur if it *has* gone away. At various times, you may for any number of reasons want to seek medical care for your PMS.

- You may want confirmation that you have PMS or reassurance that you do not have some other problem. Although increasing numbers of doctors and other health care providers are learning about PMS, the well-read woman with PMS may know more than her health care providers about what PMS is and how it can be treated. No other conditions mimic PMS, which is to say that cyclic premenstrual symptoms constitute PMS.
- Emotional and physical symptoms of PMS may be frightening. If you are afraid of losing control or are having severe physical problems such as headaches or asthma, you may need medical assistance in dealing with those symptoms.
- You may have tried self-help methods without success or without adequate success and may now want to go on to medically prescribed treatments.
- You may feel unable to cope with the work and discipline of self-help methods. PMS can leave you so worn out that you cannot contemplate a change of diet or cannot exercise regularly on your own. In that case

you may want to begin medications, sometimes with the hope that after a period of successful treatment you can try other methods.

Finding adequate medical care for this condition can be difficult depending on the availability of knowledgeable practitioners and your financial resources. PMS was first treated in this country in clinics devoted entirely to the treatment of PMS. Slowly the medical profession has begun to accept the validity of PMS, and women can more easily obtain help from their regular medical sources.

However, physicians still have a lot of fear in recognizing and treating PMS. Some of their resistance is quite inconsistent with their attitudes toward other illnesses and treatments. They use progesterone for infertility with less hesitation than for PMS, although they are thus exposing a woman *and* her fetus to the drug. They use Depo-Provera (a progestogen) in the face of extensive hearings questioning its safety. And of course they remove uteruses and ovaries with little hesitation in spite of the obvious risks and no proof of the effectiveness of this treatment for PMS.

In medical training, "women's complaints" are often the butt of teaching jokes. Doctors get used to ignoring them, laughing at them, discounting their validity. Studies have shown that when women and men go to doctors with the same problems, the complaints of the men are taken more seriously. The medical profession's attitudes toward PMS are not restricted to male physicians. The tendency to ignore women's complaints is often determined more by our indoctrination than by our gender. Female doctors often react to PMS with the same denial or lack of sensitivity as male doctors. Women need to consider these factors as they seek and assess medical care for their PMS.

In no health situation should you simply approach your physician or other health care provider and say, "Fix me." That is especially true in PMS, where the consumer may know more about the subject than the doctor and where many of the treatments are experimental and may require extreme life-style changes.

Also, as in any health situation, your own attitudes partly influence how you are treated. This is tricky in PMS, where many women come to a physician with vulnerability about being believed, with gratitude for any attention or help, but also with many resentments about past experiences seeking help. Coming to terms with PMS often involves going through stages of anger, acceptance, blaming all your troubles on PMS, a sense of betrayal by your own body, anger about previous unsuccessful treatments, anger at previous practitioners, and unrealistic expectations. All of these are normal reactions to the discovery of PMS or validation of the difficulties that have long been experienced. Recognition of their presence may make obtaining future help easier and more fruitful.

A woman considering going to a PMS clinic should consider the following:

COST: Clinics tend to charge in the range of $300 to $700 for an initial evaluation. This has sometimes included and other times been in addition to the expense of laboratory and psychological testing. Often when women call they are told the cost is less than it really is because of the assumption that insurance will cover the cost of laboratory testing. Since not everyone has insurance and since not all insurance covers all testing, inquire about lab costs in advance.

TESTING: There are no laboratory or psychological tests diagnostic for PMS. There have been some suggestions of tests that might be useful, but none have been confirmed as reliably valid. Often both lab and psychological tests are being done for research, in which case you should be so informed. Often the tests you will take are not used to diagnose PMS but to diagnose or rule out other disorders.

AVAILABILITY: Make sure there is someone from the clinic available at all times. This need not be a physician. Often the nurses working in PMS are as knowledgeable as physicians, but you should know when someone is available and who that person is.

TREATMENTS: Some clinics put major emphasis on drug treatments rather than self-help programs. Dietary and life-style counseling is more time-consuming and costly to provide. The same factors are present in many other medical facilities.

In looking for an individual doctor or nurse practitioner, you need to consider these guidelines as well as some specific questions you might ask. There are no clear-cut answers to these questions, but they are valid and important to raise and will tell you a lot about the practitioner:

1. What causes PMS? The answer to this will tell you much about this person's attitudes about both PMS and women's problems.

2. What are the possible therapies for PMS? Look for breadth of answers.

3. Which ones has he/she used and why?

4. What is this practitioner's favorite, or the one with which he/she is most successful?

5. What are the risks of each treatment?

6. What are the costs of each treatment?

SOME NO-NO'S:

- Hysterectomy: This has often been found to make PMS worse. In addition, depression often follows hysterectomy, and this is especially dangerous for women with premenstrual depression.

   After a radical hysterectomy my PMS symptoms came back much worse than they had been. I had severe headaches [migraine included], arthritic type pains in my back, hip, and shoulders, breast pain and swelling, severe fluid retention which had caused high blood pressure, tension, depression, severe mood swings, and insomnia.

- Provera and Depo-Provera: Depo-Provera is a long-acting form of Provera, a progestogen often confused with the natural progesterone and given for PMS. Depo-Provera, given as an injection to stop ovulation and the menstrual period for one to several months, often depresses women. If there is an untoward reaction to the drug, it takes weeks or months to get it out of the body. It also has some potentially dangerous long-term effects. Provera is given by pill form. So if a doctor says you are getting progesterone by pill, it is not progesterone.
- Electroconvulsive therapy (shock treatment): In some places this radical treatment is being used for PMS. The depression of PMS ends with

the menses. ECT has many long-term serious effects on memory and thinking ability. It has not been shown to be of any use in PMS.
• Tranquilizers:

> *I consulted an endocrinologist who gave me tranquiliz-*
> *ers and said I was okay.*

Tranquilizers can at times be useful for acute anxiety, but they are addicting and sedating. They do not leave a woman feeling well, but rather suppressed.
• Losing or gaining weight: Neither will result in a lessening of PMS. The pressure to lose weight may increase stress and create states of temporary starvation, and therefore increase premenstrual symptoms. Being under pressure to lose weight can make the bloating psychologically more devastating.
• Miscellaneous advice: Getting or giving up a job, getting married or unmarried, having children, etc. While any of these may be what you eventually want to do in the course of improving your life and health, beware of such pat solutions for PMS. None of them by themselves is an answer.

As you search for help with your PMS, take your charts with you and believe in your own story, your own experience, your own past. Look to professionals for their skills and guidance, but not necessarily for validation of your own truths.

In every person there is a drive toward health. Some healing can be accomplished on your own, some with the help of others, both friends and professionals. It is that basic self-healing energy, though, that must be called on by women and those who are helping them in the treatment of phenomena related to the menstrual cycle.

Selected Bibliography

Airola, Paavo. *Hypoglycemia: A Better Approach.* Phoenix, AZ: Health Plus, Publishers, 1977
Easily understood explanations of hypoglycemia in its various forms. One of the most balanced hypoglycemic diets, but it is vegetarian and some foods listed may be unfamiliar.

Bennett, William, and Joel Gurin. *The Dieter's Dilemma.* New York: Basic Books, 1982
Useful to women with PMS trying to lose weight without fasting or stringent dieting. Excellent discussion of body size.

Boston Women's Health Book Collective. *The New Our Bodies, Ourselves.* New York: Simon and Schuster, 1985
A classic in women's health, now expanded and updated. Essential reading for any woman wanting to learn more about her body.

Capacchione, Lucia. *The Creative Journal.* Athens, OH: Swallow Press, 1979
An excellent collection of journal exercises that use writing and drawing for self-awareness.

Capelan, Rachel. *How to Hypnotize Yourself and Others.* New York: Fell, Frederick, 1981
A simple how-to book, especially useful for habit breaking.

Carrington, Patricia. Freedom in Meditation, (Second Edition) Kendall Park, NJ: Pace Educational Systems, 1984 (By mail order from Pace—see Resources).
Comprehensive discussion of meditation, its history and current uses. Detailed instruction and guidelines on how to meditate.
———. *Releasing.* New York: William Morrow, 1984.

An excellent "how to let go" of self-defeating involvement with particular people or problems in your life. Step-by-step instructions to relieve stress and tension.

Dalton, Katharina. *Once a Month.* Claremont, CA: Hunter House, 1979, 1983. *Dr. Dalton's classic work on PMS broke the silence on this disorder. Dr. Dalton sees women purely as victims of their bodies and men as victims of their women. Progesterone is described as the single solution to PMS.*

————. *The Premenstrual Syndrome and Progesterone Therapy.* Chicago: Year Book Medical Pubs., 1977. *For medical practitioners, a discussion of progesterone and a guide to its use.*

Dan, Alice J., Effie A. Graham, and Carol P. Beecher, eds. *The Menstrual Cycle,* Vol. 1, New York: Springer, 1980. *A valuable collection of papers by scholars in different disciplines. Work is often critical of previous research and theory about the menstrual cycle.*

Debrovner, C., ed. *Premenstrual Tension.* New York: Human Sciences Press, 1982. *Written for professionals, this book contains various approaches to PMS treatment.*

Edwards, Betty. *Drawing on the Right Side of the Brain.* Los Angeles: J.P. Tarcher, 1979. *This book teaches you how to draw and enjoy it even if you feel you have little talent. Useful for stress reduction and self-awareness.*

Federation of Feminist Women's Health Centers. *How to Stay Out of the Gynecologist's Office.* Los Angeles: Women to Women Publications, 1981.

————. *A New View of a Woman's Body.* New York: Simon and Schuster, 1981. *These two books present radical and important descriptions of women's bodies and women's health care.*

Frankl, Viktor E. *The Unheard Cry for Meaning.* New York: Simon and Schuster, 1978. *A book about identity and meaning that can be very useful for women with PMS.*

Gendlin, Eugene. *Focusing.* New York: Everest House, 1973. *A technique to identify and change the way your personal problems manifest themselves in your body.*

Golub, Sharon, ed. *Lifting the Curse of Menstruation.* New York: Haworth Press, 1983. *Papers reviewing current literature, and challenging researchers' assumptions about the role of the menstrual cycle in women's lives.*

Hittleman, Richard. *Yoga Twenty-Eight-Day Exercise Plan.* New York: Workman, 1969 *Amply illustrated yoga exercises directed toward relieving many types of physical tension.*

————. *Yoga for Health.* New York: Ballantine Books, 1983 *Easy-to-follow instructions for the beginner at yoga. Useful nutritional information and recipes, good clear illustrations.*

Krieger, Dolores. *The Therapeutic Touch.* Englewood Cliffs, NJ: Prentice-Hall, 1979

Clear and concise, this book describes therapeutic touch as a method of healing and shows how to apply it.

Lark, Susan M. *Premenstrual Syndrome Self-Help Book.* Los Angeles: Forman Publishing, 1984
A self-help approach with diet, exercise, and acupressure massage.

Lauersen, Niels H., and Eileen Stukane. *Premenstrual Syndrome and You.* New York: Simon and Schuster, 1983
A good beginning book for understanding PMS. Contains a list of PMS resources.

Lever, Judy, and Brian Haynes. *Premenstrual Tension.* New York: McGraw-Hill, 1981
An early discussion of PMS, this contains some good basic information but is not as complete as later books.

Namikoshi, Toru. *Shiatsu Therapy.* New York: Japan Publications, 1977
A discussion of principles of Shiatsu therapy and problems it will alleviate.

Nofziger, Margaret. *A Cooperative Method of Natural Birth Control.* Summertown, TN: Book Publishing Company, 1976
Excellent how-to book for charting ovulation both by basal body temperature and changes in cervical mucus.

Norris, Ronald V., with Colleen Sullivan. *PMS: Premenstrual Syndrome.* New York: Rawson Wade, 1983
Informative review of PMS, including its history. Contains some useful suggestions about diagnosis and treatment.

Ojeda, Linda. *Exclusively Female.* Claremont, CA: Hunter House, 1983
Concise information on diet and vitamins for menstrual irregularities, dysmenorrhea and premenstrual syndrome.

Orbach, Susie. *Fat Is a Feminist Issue II.* New York: Berkley, 1982
A program for compulsive eating. Useful to women whose PMS includes loss of control over eating.

Popenoe, Cris. *Wellness.* New York: Random House, 1977
Contains hundreds of descriptions of books about health, nutrition, exercise, and alternative healing methods. See also the listing for the Yes! Bookshop under Resources for Books and Tapes.

Reitz, Rosetta. *Menopause: A Positive Approach.* New York: Penguin Books, 1979
An excellent book about physiological and psychological changes in menopause.

Shaffer, Martin. *Life After Stress.* Chicago: Contemporary Books, 1983
A good basic book explaining how to assess stress and relieve it.

van Keep, Pieter A., and Wulf H. Utian, eds. *The Premenstrual Syndrome.* Lancaster, Eng.: MTP Press Limited, 1981
The proceedings of a workshop held during the Sixth International Congress of Obstetrics and Gynecology, Berlin, September 1980. Interesting scientific papers with panel member discussions.

Woolfolk, Robert I., and Frank C. Richardson. *Stress, Sanity, and Survival.* New York: New American Library, 1979
An excellent primer on reducing stress.

Cookbooks

Here are some cookbooks whose recipes are generally consistent with a PMS diet. Note that some recipes in all these cookbooks include sugar substitutes such as honey, molasses, or maple syrup, all of which should be avoided on a PMS diet.

Airola, Paavo. *The Airola Diet and Cookbook.* Phoenix, AZ: Health Plus, Publishers, 1981

Ewald, Ellen Buchman. *Recipes for a Small Planet.* New York: Ballantine Books, 1975

Goldbeck, Nikki and David. *American Wholefoods Cuisine.* New York: New American Library, 1983.

Hewitt, Jean. *The New York Times New Natural Foods Cookbook.* New York: Times Books, 1982

Katzen, Mollie. *Moosewood Cookbook.* Berkeley, CA: Ten Speed Press, 1977

Lappé, Frances Moore. *Diet for a Small Planet.* New York: Ballantine Books, 1982

Robertson, Laurel, Carol Flinders, and Bronwen Godfrey. *Laurel's Kitchen.* Petaluma, Calif.: Nilgiri Press, 1976

Thomas, Anna. *The Vegetarian Epicure.* New York: Vintage Books, 1972

Thomas, Anna. *The Vegetarian Epicure, Book Two.* New York: Alfred A. Knopf, 1978

Resources for Books and Tapes

Pace Educational Systems, Inc.
P.O. Box 113
Kendall Park, NJ 08824

Distributes books, cassettes and training materials by Dr. Patricia Carrington, an authority on stress reduction methods.

The Soundworks, Inc.
911 North Fillmore Street
Arlington, VA 22201
800-422-0111

Distributes a wide variety of cassettes dealing with health, stress, relationships, and the plight of the universe.

Yes! Bookshop
1035 31st Street N.W.
Washington, DC 20007

This store distributes books on health care, stress reduction, alternative therapies, and nutrition (including cookbooks). See also the listing for Wellness *by Cris Popenoe in the Selected Bibliography.*

Food Sources

Here are two mail-order companies that stock foods compatible with the PMS diet.

Bioforce of America, Ltd.
21 West Mall
Plainview, NY 11803

This company sells natural health products from Switzerland. Their noncaffeine coffee-like product Bambu is sold in handy individual packets as well as in regular containers.

Walnut Acres
Penns Creek, PA 17862

Excellent source of organic and whole-grain foods without preservatives. Good for canned goods, whole-grain flour, bread mixes, pastas, nuts, grain, herbs and spices, as well as cookbooks.

PMS Resources

PMS Action
P.O. Box 19669
Irvine, CA 92713
714-752-6355

A national nonprofit organization committed to helping women become informed, active health consumers. They provide educational material that consists of information on PMS symptoms, support groups, treatment options and self-help techniques. PMS Action conducts professional training programs and refers women to physicians and other health practitioners throughout the United States. They also publish a newsletter, The PMS Connection.

The National PMS Society
3514 University Drive, Suite 5
Durham, NC 27707
919-489-6577

A nonprofit organization whose membership is made up of physicians, pharmacists, nurse practitioners, and lay people. The PMS Society's stated purposes are: (1) to educate the public and professionals; (2) to assist PMS sufferers by referrals, a newsletter, support groups, hot lines, and public meetings; (3) to raise money for PMS research.

Madison Pharmacy Associates, Inc.
1603 Monroe Street, Box 9641
Madison, WI 53715
608-257-7046, 1-800-588-7046 (outside Wisconsin)

One of the first sources of progesterone in the United States, they continue to mail-order progesterone, vitamins, medications, and reading materials useful for PMS. The staff is available to physicians and pharmacists as well as lay people desiring information about PMS and its treatment.

SYMPTOMS   INITIALS

1. ——————————————————————   ——————

2. ——————————————————————   ——————   Menstruation:

3. ——————————————————————   ——————   Date charting began: ——————————————

MONTHS

1								
2								
3								
4								
5								
6								
7								
8								
9								
10								
11								
12								
13								
14								
15								
16								
17								
18								
19								
20								
21								
22								
23								
24								
25								
26								
27								
28								
29								
30								
31								

SYMPTOMS   INITIALS

1. ———————————————————   ————

2. ———————————————————   ————   Menstruation:

3. ———————————————————   ————   Date charting began: ——————————

MONTHS

1								
2								
3								
4								
5								
6								
7								
8								
9								
10								
11								
12								
13								
14								
15								
16								
17								
18								
19								
20								
21								
22								
23								
24								
25								
26								
27								
28								
29								
30								
31								

Exercise Journal

EXERCISE I LIKE	EXERCISE TO RETRY	EXERCISE I ALWAYS WANTED TO TRY

FIVE EXERCISES TO TRY THIS MONTH

1. Exercise _____ How I will do it _____
   _____

2. Exercise _____ How I will do it _____
   _____

3. Exercise _____ How I will do it _____
   _____

4. Exercise _____ How I will do it _____
   _____

5. Exercise _____ How I will do it _____
   _____

FILL-IN EXERCISES While I am trying new forms of exercise I will use the following exercises on a daily basis so that each day I do something.

_____

_____

_____

Weekly Exercise Journal

Use this form to keep track of the exercises you are doing. It will be interesting to see how, over time, your ability and pleasure increase.

Week of _____

	S	M	T	W	T	F	S
EXERCISE							
TIME OF DAY							
HOW LONG							
HOW IT FELT							
WHAT NEEDS TO BE CHANGED							

Bad Day Report

DATE _____   LAST PERIOD _____

DAY OF CYCLE _____

What happened?

Foods eaten (note also any long stretches without eating):

Exercise:

Current stresses:

Review of the day several days later: How does the day look in retro-spect? Are issues raised that still may be important? Was the diet that day a healthy one? What have you learned?

About the Author

DR. MICHELLE HARRISON was one of the first doctors in the United States to specialize in premenstrual syndrome and is now a leading authority on the subject. Her frequent lectures and public appearances focus mainly on PMS and other women's health issues. She graduated from New York Medical College in 1967 and has had experience in family medicine, psychiatry and ob-gyn. Dr. Harrison now has a private practice devoted exclusively to premenstrual syndrome in Cambridge, Massachusetts, where she lives with her two children. She is the author of *A Woman in Residence*.